STOLEN

*How Surgical Mesh Stole Years of
Health and Dreams From Me and
Countless Others.*

by Diane Ritter-Gardner RN,BSN

Edited by Lil Barcaski

Published by: GWN Publishing
www.GWNPublishing.com

Cover Design: Kristina Conatser

ISBN: 978-1-959608-80-6

DEDICATION

This book is dedicated to all of humanity; all people, women or men, some of whom may be ill and do not know why. And to all seeking healthcare. We deserve kindness and truth about our bodies and our psyches'. We have the right to know everything that will benefit or impair the quality of our lives, giving us the greatest gift of all, a choice!

And especially to women.

Women who are surviving with polypropylene mesh inside of them now or even after its attempt to be removed, as in my case.

This book is for us.

AFTER A WHILE

After a while you learn the subtle difference
between holding a hand and chaining a soul,
and you learn that love doesn't mean leaning
and company doesn't always mean security.

And you begin to learn that kisses aren't contracts
and presents aren't promises.

And you begin to accept your defeats with your head up
and your eyes ahead,
with the grace of a woman, not the grief of a child.

And you learn to build all your roads on today,
because tomorrow's ground is too uncertain for plans
and futures have a way of falling down in mid-flight.

After a while you learn that even sunshine burns
if you get too much
so you plant your own garden
and decorate your own soul,
instead of waiting for someone to bring you flowers.

And you learn that you really can endure,
you really are strong,
you really have worth,
and you learn,
and you learn,
with every goodbye, you learn.

By: Veronica A. Shoffstall

TABLE OF CONTENTS

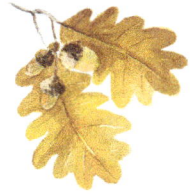

INTRODUCTION

I have been a registered nurse for 43 years and have seen a lot of life and a lot of death. Some at work as a nurse and some very close to home. I believe that before polypropylene mesh was implanted into my body, I was an extraordinary woman. I survived through some extremely tough times—the sudden death of my spouse when I was 33 with three young daughters and sudden brain surgery after years of severe headaches, to name two.

The most devastating issue that I have been dealing with for over 14 years has caused me and most likely millions of other people, particularly women, the most physical and emotional pain ever. I am thankful that I know enough about my body that I did not give up *on myself*. If I had, I believe I would have died.

In this book, I am going to tell you about the many hoops I had to jump through to finally realize what was literally taking my life from me. I am writing this book in hopes, that if you are experiencing some of what I did, you will look at my journey, through the healthcare system of today, and know that not all doctors or surgeons have the answer to all issues. They certainly did not have the answers for me. I want you to know that it is not only okay to ask questions, before you make medical decisions about your body, but it is essential that you do. My hope is that you will be fully involved in your healthcare, hopefully preventing the mishaps that have stolen my life, *as it should be*, from me.

The title "STOLEN" reflects the things that were and still are being stolen from my life. This is, in part, because of the many areas of our healthcare system which are failing. I have encountered overly confident and perhaps under informed practitioners, several of whom were either afraid to, or simply would not prescribe, pain medicine to me; medication that I have been on for years. Other physicians, including primary care physicians, were not very comfortable prescribing controlled substances and so they were sending people, me included, to "pain specialists." No doubt they were all worried about the crackdown on opioids, known in Florida at that time (2010-2014,) as the "Oxycontin express", but at the same time, not taking into consideration that some people are suffering with chronic pain. I needed these medications and by abruptly withholding them from me or anyone else in my circumstance, it could cause devastating withdrawal symptoms even up to the point of death. I do not feel that I was abusing drugs. My PCP was prescribing me Tramadol, which I still take today. I was not going from doctor to doctor asking for controlled substances. *Suddenly* withholding certain medications from patients, who have built up a medically necessary dependence on them (or not), can put their life at risk. I was fortunate that my PCP knew me and was willing to take care of me. She was just as frustrated as I was regarding my continued ever-increasing pain.

Polypropylene Mesh:

This mesh remained in my body for five years. According to "Drug watch," Polypropylene Mesh is associated with several serious hernia mesh complications, particularly in men. In my opinion *this alone makes mesh not conducive to long-term* placement in the human body. Mesh erodes, attaches, crimps, and destroys tissue. And yet, mesh continues to be used today, particularly in middle-aged women needing gynecologic surgeries, like hysterectomies, or relief from stress urinary incontinence or perhaps repair of the many of the prolapses affecting women today. In my book, I will take you through some of what I have experienced with hope that it helps you when making your medical choices.

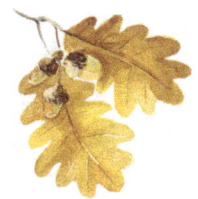

FIRST, I WANT YOU TO KNOW ABOUT MY YOUNGER YEARS

I was born in a time when babies played with wooden beads on a sting, and had blankets, bottles, and stuffed animals in their crib. Balloons at birthday parties were not considered dangerous due to the choking hazard should a child suck it into their lungs while trying to blow it up. They even put beaded bracelets on newborns. That would never happen today. They got my last name wrong on the first one. I'm surprised they replaced it.

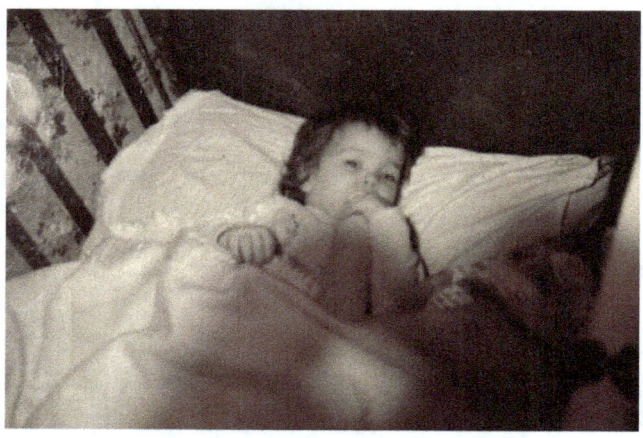

Me as a baby with my bottle

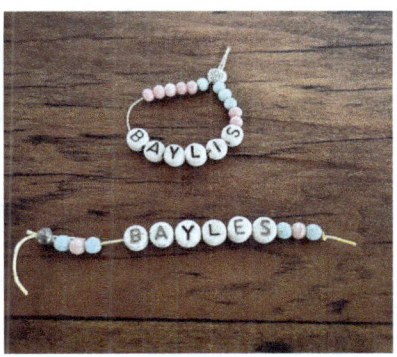

Chockable baby bracelet

I was brought up in the city, just outside of Boston. My childhood was normal for a city kid in the 1960s, until age eight, when I walked alone to the "Elliot Market." On my way home I was supposed to go to the crosswalk at the corner, where, coincidentally, my dad was sitting in his car at a red light. But in all my excitement of getting my new Superball, I tried to cross sooner and stepped behind a large truck right onto the street.

All I remember is looking to the right and seeing a black car coming toward me. I was in the middle of the road, and I could not hear any sounds, no horns, no voices. I could not move! All I saw was the car. The next thing I remember was waking up to my dad's voice. I tried to open my eyes but saw nothing, I could feel a warm fluid running down my face... blood. I still think of this trauma too often.

Later, my dad told me that once I was hit by the car, I was thrown approximately 100 feet and landed on my head. As an emergency room nurse, I know that the head bleeds well! I also fractured my skull. My dad went into what I call "cop mode." He didn't realize it was me at first. He would have helped anyone.

I remember hearing the sirens of the ambulance and my distraught mother screaming behind the stretcher as I was pushed down the hospital hallway. I cannot imagine her anguish. I woke up to the pain of a spinal tap needle and seeing only a glass wall. Then, apparently days later, I woke up on the other side of that glass wall. I told my mother I wanted to go home. She contacted the doctor, and I went home in a cab with two huge black eyes, not remembering any other specifics to this day. I wish I had asked more questions of my parents before they passed away. I was so lucky to be alive but too young to even realize it. It turned out the man driving the car was my brother's teacher. Apparently, he visited me in the hospital and brought me another Superball. To this day, I cringe when I see Superballs in stores.

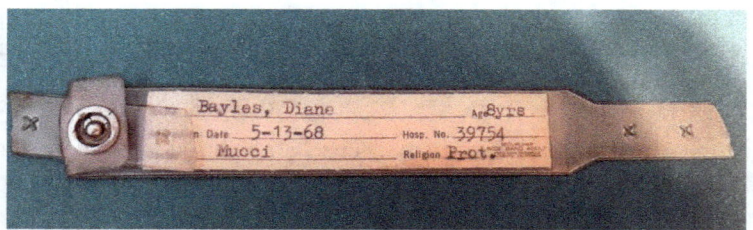

My hospital ID bracelet for my accident

Other than this excruciatingly, traumatic experience, my childhood was like other kids of this generation. I was voted "most popular" in 6th grade. *Crazy that they even did such a thing.* I was active in student council, played sports, and had many friends. Academically, I was a good student, getting A's and B's throughout all my education.

I had one more head injury as a kid when a neighbor kid threw a brick at me! Hitting me, *yep, you guessed it,* in the head! I still have the scar. Another taxi ride to the emergency room. This time it was a concussion, stitches, and another black eye. *This wasn't the end of my headaches.*

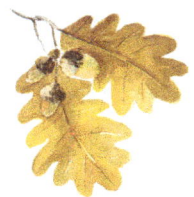

FROM CITY LIFE TO
COUNTRY LIFE

When I was 15 years old, my dad, now promoted to SGT, accepted a transfer within the MDC. We moved to the geographical center of Massachusetts, home to Boston's water supply, the Quabbin Reservoir in Hardwick, Massachusetts. This picturesque body of water, and its surrounding watershed was the result of flooding several towns and then the building of two huge dams. It is a beautiful body of water closed off to the public other than some picnic areas and seasonal fishing behind specific gates. The MDC (Metropolitan District Commission) polices this land, so off to the country we moved. It was a drastic change for everyone. My brothers were out of the picture at this point. We moved to Hardwick until the "state-owned" house on the other side of the reservoir was available.

My late husband, Ernest Ritter II, or "Ritter" as I called him, lived in Hardwick. When my sister and I checked into the office on our first day of school, Ritter happened to be volunteering. Not only was he very attentive to us, but he also just happened to be on the same bus route and offered to meet us after school and guide us to the bus. Being city girls, my sister and I had never taken a school bus before. So, we accepted his offer. It was at least an hour to get to school for us and an hour back with many stops. This was rural Massachusetts!

Ritter drew attention to himself by telling jokes, and generally being the "bus clown." I thought he was ridiculous.

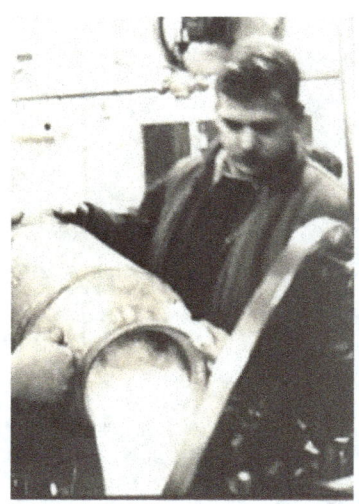

His family's business processed and delivered milk and other dairy products to people's front porches in the wee hours of the morning. *Yes, they delivered very early, in glass bottles*, where milk boxes sat. The little house my parents rented was about 15 miles out of town, *in the "sticks."*

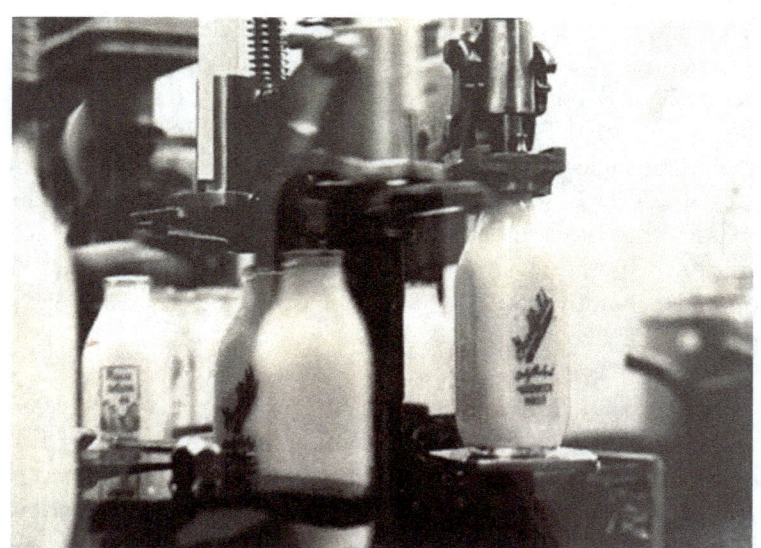

Milk processing

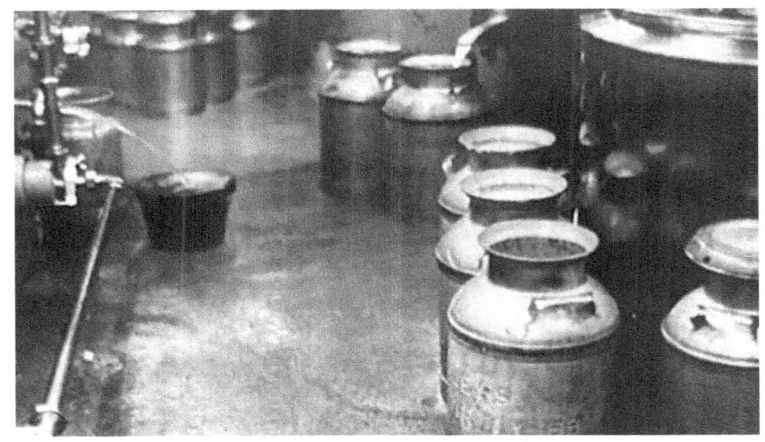

Milk cans

Ritter tried many ways to get my attention, but the craziest was when he stopped at our house with a pint of fresh cream for my mother, saying that it would not last the ride back to the dairy. *He was driving a refrigerated delivery truck.* I accepted this gift knowing that he would have to return to collect the glass bottle. *Quite the ploy!* He also sent me daisies and had the florist sign the card "guess who?" And then, he showed up on my doorstep with flowers on May 1st, *May Day.* I had never heard of this tradition. In 1977 he got up the nerve to propose at dinner, in the same Inn where his parents had their wedding reception. We got married on July 14, 1979. It was the hottest day of the summer and with all his fraternity brothers in attendance. All of the wedding party got thrown in the pool except for me!

Ritter joined ROTC in high School already knowing he would join Army ROTC in College. He got degrees in animal husbandry and business administration.

He and I made a deal that if we were still in the Army at the 10-year mark, we would stay in for the long haul of 20 years. Discussing our possible retirement from the Army, Ritter expressed wanting to raise Christmas trees for his favorite holiday and to have an ice cream stand in the summer. He loved making homemade ice cream for our girls' birthdays.

Believe me, an Army wife's job is never done! I bought this poster (right) at one of our monthly wives' club meetings. The artist was there, so I got it signed. It shows some of the many "jobs" of a military wife. We were expected to join in gatherings such as military balls, which were fun. We just had to find a babysitter. I not only took care of my own kids but military family's kids too. The military exists as one big family. I stood by my soldier for award ceremonies and promotions, kept supper warm for the many late nights, and I was a single parent when Ritter went "down range." I did my share of ironing uniforms and sewing on patches. They have Velcro now! Lucky ducks. I entertained sometimes without warning, and I tried to keep things in order at home for these surprise visitors. All these things and so much more. I also happen to be a military mother. Two of my daughters are in the military, both nurses, one Army and one Air Force. My third daughter supports her sisters wholeheartedly and she is a proud military daughter and sister.

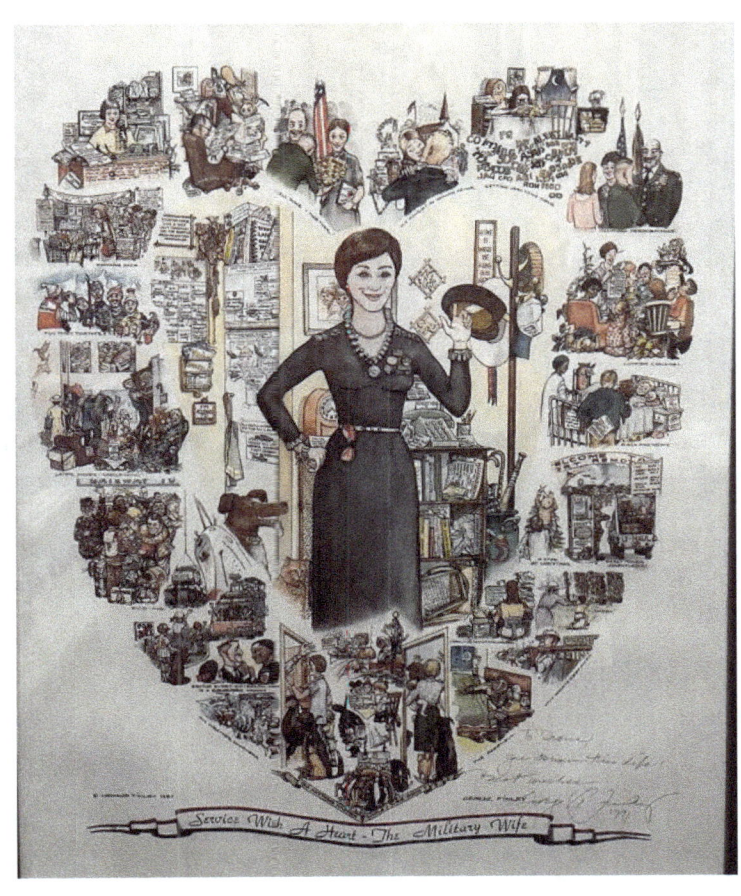

Service with a heart

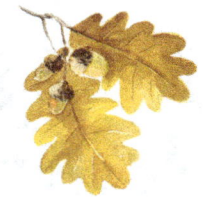

WE'RE IN THE ARMY NOW

R itter chose his first tour as a "hardship tour" to Korea, unaccompanied. I was a senior in nursing school, and we got married that year in July. Once home from Korea, (he always seemed to get a "Christmas drop" and so, most years we were home by Christmas), Ritter went to Ft Sill, Oklahoma, "home of the artillery," for his basic training.

Our first tour together was in Ft Carson, Colorado. I worked emergency in a trauma 1 hospital. Many stabbings, gunshot wounds, rape victims, and their accused attackers were brought in. In 1981 while working on a police officer who had been stabbed in the chest, I began to bleed vaginally. Not a lot, but enough for concern. I called my OB-GYN doctor. Meanwhile, the ER doctor cracked the police officer's chest, and someone performed internal compressions. We tried resuscitating him for a long time. *He was a friend, as was all the police force.*

I did a pregnancy test, and it was positive. I decided to leave the job, go put my feet up until the bleeding stopped, which eventually it did. My first two daughters were born at that hospital in "The Springs" in 1982 and 1984. My third daughter was born in Brunswick, Maine in 1987. A true "Maine-a." Between 1979, the year of our marriage, and 1992, the year of his death, Ritter moved 12 times. This included his hardship tour to Korea, and basic training. During these years, I had nine different nursing jobs. I never had any trouble finding a position in nursing.

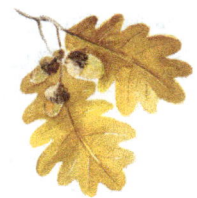

MY EXTRAORDINARY EXPERIENCES

To be extraordinary, you must be able to endure those things in life that you don't think you can. I see myself as a kind person. I am reliable and trustworthy. To live up to being extraordinary, I look back on my profession as a registered nurse, as well as raising three truly extraordinary daughters mostly on my own after Ritter passed away.

Experiences in My Nursing Positions

Staying with a mother, crying with her, after an unsuccessful resuscitation of her only child—a son—who got hit by a pickup truck crossing the street to see a dead cat. I remember his right arm hanging limp over the side of the stretcher. It was so hard for all involved. What can you say or do for a parent who loses a child? I had no words. There is no way to fill that void.

To jump on a patient who is bleeding so fast you have no time for gloves during the AIDS (acquired immunodeficiency syndrome) epidemic when universal precautions were just getting started. Certain instincts are hard to un-learn.

Supporting the family and fiancé of a young woman who went to surgery for a simple ovarian cyst removal. They never got to the surgery because she reacted so badly to the anesthetic that her larynx spasmed, blocking her airway. The code team could not break the spasm or re-open her airway in time. She already had significant loss of brain function when they wheeled her into the ICU, where I was the team leader. I later learned she passed away in a nursing home sometime after. The stories can go on and on.

My nursing experience has been in many areas. I started out in the emergency department of the hospital my nursing school was affiliated with. The challenge was being ready to help anyone who came through the doors. I got my ACLS (advanced cardiac life support) certification. I also taught ACLS for a while. There are crazy things that go on in the emergency department. Emergency room staff and the local police department work together, helping each other in various situations. This usually includes some chatting and a cup of coffee. I think there is an unspoken respect between the two professions. Because my dad was a police officer, I always enjoyed sharing appropriate stories with the local PD.

My sister is an emergency room nurse and not long ago when she got off her shift, she found a newborn baby in a box on the ground right next to her car. This brand-new baby boy had his umbilical cord still attached. In the United States, as well as Puerto Rico, Guam, and the District of Columbia there is a "safe haven" law which allows mothers or anyone to bring an infant to an emergency department, or other public buildings. I believe most nurses and other public servants would be more than happy to take an infant into a "safe haven." Thankfully, this newborn was fine. Also in Colorado, when I was pregnant and had stopped bleeding, I worked at a family practice clinic. I really enjoyed the teaching I could do on a basic level for all patients. I also started a blood pressure clinic in which we took everyone's blood pressure, went over causes and treatment of hypertension.

Our next "stop" was a quick school In Georgia, our middle daughter was so young, and Ritter was only there for a six-month course, so we rented a house. I joined the YWCA so I could swim for exercise, and I volunteered at the military hospital. Once in Maine, both in Bangor and Brunswick, I worked at emergency departments of small hospitals in each city (two years each.) In the ED of SJH in Bangor, a construction guy casually walked in with his buddy who had a one-and-a-half-inch nail in his head. It was driven right into his temple. It must have missed all vital organs because he was stable for transport to EMMC. There was always excitement, no matter how small the department.

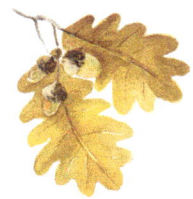

THE BEST YEAR OF OUR LIFE

When Ritter was given orders to Leavenworth for *"the best year of his life and ours,"* we wives were skeptical. In the end, I still have fond memories of antiquing with Ritter and my BFF, Fatty.

At Fort Leavenworth, a one-year school for Ritter, I worked for a miserable five months of 12hr nights, 7pm to 7am, until my family, mostly Ritter, begged me to stop. I guess I got a bit sleep-deprived, tired of caring for prisoners, brought in the middle of the night by the guards. I was always very grumpy. I learned that working nights is not for me. The remainder of the time, I took some craft classes, took my girls to craft classes, collected a lot of cool antiques and filled in for the school nurse for a month or so. It truly was a wonderful year, even if we were surrounded by two huge penitentiaries.

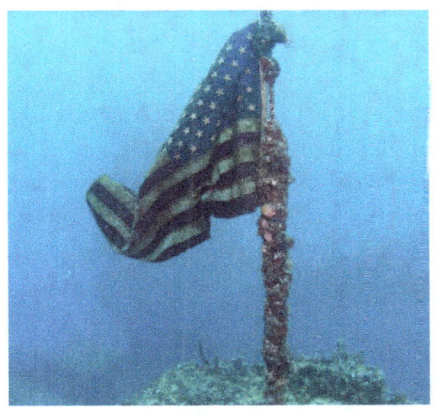

Underwater dive flag

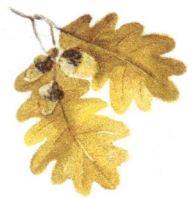

MY LIFE FLIPPED UPSIDE DOWN, OVERSEAS

From Kansas, it was off to Germany where I managed a six bed PACU (recovery room) at the military hospital. This turned out to be a fiasco. I had two LPNs working for me. One was a military SGT with a poor attitude and the other a new hire civilian. I documented every move this "LPN" took. She had put a child's life in danger, and I was glad to have, at least, terminated her employment just before my husband, Ritter, was tragically killed in a head on collision. I did not choose her as my hire. My boss did. I really don't think she was even a nurse. Then none of this mattered as my life was about to make a tragic turn.

Ritter rose to the rank of Major while we were stationed in Germany and at the two-year mark, he became the executive officer of a field artillery battalion. This position was the reason we were there. It was why he had attended CGSC (Command and General Staff College) at Ft Leavenworth, Kansas. Right after he graduated from this year long class, we got orders to Würzburg, Germany.

Desert Storm had broken out, keeping Ritter very busy. After two years of working hard as the materials readiness officer for supplies going to Saudi Arabia, preparing and waiting for his promotion, he was advanced to the XO position he had been groomed for. About one month into that new assignment, Ritter fell asleep while driving causing the collision that took his life. No-one else was injured. This catastrophic event left me with our three precious girls, then ages ten, eight, and four, a boat load of responsibilities, many lost dreams and a broken heart that I never would have ever anticipated.

Our "military family" was extremely supportive. I was never left alone. It so happened that when Ritter died, our oldest daughter, H, was at Euro Disney with the girl scouts. Ritter's commander, Col. B, who is family to us now, offered to have a helicopter fly to Paris and get H right away. I chose to let her finish the trip. Our middle daughter was at a sleepover nearby with her best friend. There was no problem extending that for another couple of days. My baby, E, then four years old, fell asleep in my bed that night before R went missing. I am sure that she sensed the turmoil suddenly thrust upon me and ultimately all of us. She did, however, go when someone came and took her for play time and an overnight. The night before the accident, according to Ritter's commander and our now adored family friend, Major Gen.L.B (ret), he had walked Ritter home after work that evening. A few of the guys were hanging around outside and so, after Ritter changed his clothes, he went back out and tried to get the guys to go get something to eat. He had also mentioned that he had carried E to her own bed before he drove off seeking food. We both always tried to put the girls back in their own beds if they wandered into ours in the middle of night. That night Ritter held E in his arms for the last time, on this earth.

I don't remember seeing my youngest much during that week. I don't remember a whole lot about the week in general. I think E was fine with friends since she was used to daddy being away a lot. We had a lot of friends right there on base, very close, loving friends who we still have today. I waited until H came home from Paris, then I remember sitting on my bed to tell my three girls that their daddy had died. This event and the time leading up to telling my girls is the most agonizing thing I have ever done in my life. My friends and my military family protected me from myself. Thank God I had our girls to remind me of the strength I might not have known I had and needed to muster up. I had to stop banging my head against the wall, literally. I had to be there for my daughters. I was allowed to sit with my husband's flag draped casket in the chapel for a time. There was always someone watching me. Just in case I needed anything, they were there to support me. I wore the red dress that I had purchased online for the Artillery Ball. It still hangs in my closet.

We returned to the states after the memorial service that was held for my husband at The Marne Garden on base in Würzburg, Germany. Although it was a very still day, I clearly remember Ritter's dog tags tinkling in the breeze as they hung over his "spit-shined" boots. I felt his presence that day.

My daughters had been working very hard preparing for a gymnastics meet scheduled for that weekend. I'm not sure if they were, like me, in denial, or just needed life to be "normal" for a little while longer. They had attended one day of school and were met by some callous boys, who were spreading ugly rumors about their dad. They brought all their things home and did not go back. My friend, and co-worker, Dr. BH, prescribed meds to help calm me, which made it possible for all of us to attend their gymnastics meet. I went with a friend, but felt many eyes on me. I remember the feeling of several people looking my way. I really can't say I remember much about the meet, but I wanted to escape reality, for myself and for my girls. I was being selfish, wanting to forget the real world for a little while. My daughters are all strong and self-confident, even in the midst of tragedy, young, but still proud even then, they did what they thought their dad would have wanted them to do. They did it for him.

Back to reality, in our little apartment, I remember people coming with food and I was lying on the couch with ice packs on my swollen, bloodshot eyes. I remember my boss crying while hugging me and I had no more tears. I felt guilty. It is hard to write this because I have re-lived the events of this day for 31 years. My heart breaks repeatedly inside my chest, but especially for my girls, his girls. We have kept him alive in our hearts with stories and "daddy gifts" and celebrating his birthday with ice-cream sundaes, pictures of which we all share on texts. His favorites are rum raisin and maple walnut.

My casualty assistance officer was Ritter's best friend C. He and his wife L were there for the girls and me right from the start. L took me shopping for appropriate funeral attire. I ended up with a black and white houndstooth skirt suit. That no longer hangs in my closet. L and other wonderful friends ran my household for me.

I don't remember many details of that week, before we flew back to the states. C took over the old "maid's quarters," which was just an extra room in the basement, (each officer was allotted this extra room) and made it into his temporary office. He began to do all the paperwork necessary for contacting the insurance company. He arranged for movers and packers, let the schools know my girls would not be coming back, and for so much more. He called family, arranging for certain people to not be alone when they got this horrific news. His sister went to be with Ritter's parents and my sister went to be with my mother. She loved Ritter as a son. There was more paperwork and paying off some furniture items we had recently bought at a German antique barn. The items had not been delivered yet. It boggles my mind that most widows must do this all themselves. The Army took very good care of us.

Another wonderful friend of ours, (Cpt.) SL, willingly escorted Ritter from Germany to Dover, Delaware, where military cremations are done. S stayed with Ritter the entire time. I remember that I had it in my head that I wanted S to be with Ritter every second. Now I see that S was already providing me with a sense of ease by just going with "Ritter," and I cannot imagine that he did not have a tough time of it himself. I personally have never been to a crematorium. He and his wife gave me comfort with this unexpected act of kindness. I'm not sure what the usual protocol is, but I know it took one worry off my mind knowing S was with him and stayed with him all the way to Hardwick.

C also planned the memorial service we had in Germany, and he planned our trip home. C accompanied me, my girls, and I'm guessing at least 10 duffel bags filled with bedding and stuffed animals that the girls really wanted with them. With C in charge, and "Blue Bark" orders, it was no problem to take as much as we wanted. Once back in the states, we headed to Hardwick where CPT. L had beat us home. "*Ritter*" was waiting on his parents' mantle, in an urn that I cannot recall, even though I carried him down to "his" bedroom for so many nights, before *I finally* carried him into the cemetery, where he was buried in his family plot. I do remember the 21-gun salute, and being handed Ritter's Flag. That same flag draped his casket in the hospital chapel. I put words on paper and had C read them for me at both the service in Germany and the service in Hardwick on Armed Forces Day, 1992.

Both officers, C and S, stayed and helped to plan the memorial service, which was held on Armed Forces Day in Hardwick, Massachusetts. The unspoken "rule" of "make no major decisions in your life after the death of a loved one, for at least a year" did not apply to me in these circumstances. I had to get us back to the states, get my daughters in school, find a place to live, and figure out what to do with my life. My head was swimming. I leaned heavily on God for support. On the day of his memorial service, the church billboard read,

*"The only way to take the pain out of death,
is to take the love out of life."*
AUTHOR UNKNOWN

This is so true. Less than a year went by before we moved up to Maine, where I had grown to love the lakes, the white mountains right in my daily view, and the ocean a short drive away. While living in Hardwick, I took one class toward my Baccalaureate degree, at a not-so-close-by community college. This experience of a long commute for one class helped me to decide that I needed to move to where there were some varieties of schools, for both me and the girls. I was hoping for a variety of jobs to choose from as well. I now knew that the woods of Massachusetts was not where I wanted to raise my girls.

On a drive by search for houses in the Lakes region of Sebago, Maine, I drove by the old farmhouse that was for sale. I immediately called the realtor's phone number on the sign and saw the house that day. I fell in love with it. That is where I raised my daughters, on the edge of Sebago Lake.

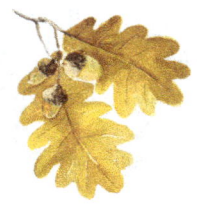

MEDICAL SURGICAL NURSING IS A YOUNG WOMEN'S SPORT

I started my RN to BSN program right away once in Maine. I also got two per diem jobs working in a nursing home and in a small medical center. Neither of these jobs really appealed to my need for autonomy or teaching. I was too busy caring for patients to teach anyone anything. Again, we were short staffed. Medical surgical nursing is hard work, a young and energetic person's job. Although I know several women and men my age or older who still run crazy in the emergency department.

I found a job I really enjoyed, working for Apria HealthCare. This job entailed me going into the hospital to meet with a patient who would be discharged home, with the intention of continuing treatment themselves or by a family member. I enjoyed teaching them and their caregiver how to either give their own IV antibiotics and manage their own pain pump among other treatments.

This was in the day of payphones; there were no cell phones yet. I would have to make my schedule and call my patient from a payphone to get directions to their home. There was no GPS yet either. I would usually start an intravenous line and teach them what the signs of infection and infiltration are. A home health nurse would take over, checking in. I managed to keep the job for about two years, but with my girl's lives being so busy, I could not drive the distances that were required to continue my job with Apria. I needed to be close enough to home should an emergency occur. Being a single parent is a lot of responsibility.

I worked several other jobs while still on the eight-year plan to my BSN at Saint Joseph's College, which conveniently was and still is about one mile from where I want to eventually settle down in retirement, on a piece of land next to the old farm. My health issues, which really slow me down, make it even more important to be able to use the facilities at SJC. Eventually, I ended up working at Orthopedic Associates, in the PACU.

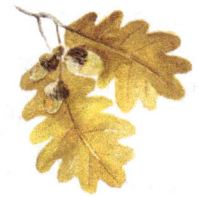

LET LOVE FIND ME

I worked at Orthopedic Associates for about four years. I had just returned from my mother's funeral in 1997. My mom needed a femoral popliteal bypass surgery, where they took a vein from one part of her body and used it to bypass the part of the artery behind the knee, where plaque had built up causing her extreme pain to walk.

Mom had a lot of health issues with high blood pressure, uncontrolled diabetes, and vascular disease in general. She had already had the carotid arteries in her neck cleaned of plaque (an endarterectomy) and she had a triple bypass surgery on her heart vessels. After the Fem-pop bypass surgery, my mom's blood pressure went sky high and despite the monitors blaring and my sister and I, both registered nurses, expressing the need for them to treat her hypertension, they did nothing.

She eventually had a stroke. They transferred her to Worcester. The last time I saw her she was not looking good, and I thought she was completely unconscious until I attempted to do mouth care on her. There was a lot of gunk on the roof of her mouth, so I put my finger in her mouth to try to dislodge and remove the built-up material. She bit my finger hard! I will never forget this message she was sending for me to *leave her alone.*

I knew she was not ready to die. She had plans to go play bingo on a bus tour the following month. She loved bingo and if her numbers were not being called, she would yell to the guy, "Shake up your balls!" She really was quite a hoot! The bingo players always knew if "Gracie" was in the house. She was opinionated and loud, but her laugh was contagious.

The stroke was too much for my mom, and she had given up. She was 68 years "young." She always said, "You are as young as you feel." We had a bingo card carved into her gravestone and a hammer for my dad. He was a great cop, but his real love was working with wood.

Driving to work my first day back from my mom's funeral, I was re-thinking my life. My dad died at age 59 and now my mom. I had also lost my husband. As a young widow of 38 years, I had been dating guys in their early 30s and realizing they were not who I would bring home to meet my girls. These guys were in a different part of their life. I prayed out loud, all the way to work that day, that God would let love find me.

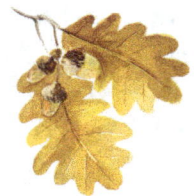

I CHECKED HIM IN,
THEN I CHECKED HIM OUT

A friend at work, MJ, had told me two weeks prior from my return to work, about a guy that she had done pre-operative testing on. This was standard operating procedure for all day surgeries. We usually did an EKG, blood work, maybe a chest x-ray, and obtained the patient's medical history. This guy was squeaky clean, and he was single. I really wasn't thinking about "this guy" on my first day back because I was sure that I had missed his surgical day having been gone for quite a while getting my mother's affairs in order.

I didn't expect God to work so fast. My husband (of 26 years now) is the guy MJ had done the pre-op on two weeks prior. That day at work, I was a "float nurse," helping where needed and so I checked in the first patient of the morning. He had torn his ACL while skiing. As I checked him in that morning, without realizing he was the guy MJ thought might be a good match for me, I immediately liked him. He was quiet, composed and easy going and best of all an easy intravenous stick. Ha! Nurses love this! He was also being picked up by his father. This was a good indication that he was single. When people ask how we met, I usually joke about how "I checked him in, and then I checked him out." He accuses me of going into the operating room and really "checking him out," *but I am too professional for that.*

It was kind of crazy, but his dad was living in the camp that Den grew up in just half of a mile down the road from me. As it turned out, Den's mom had passed away three months before my mom. His dad, F, was a carpenter like my dad and a sweet and funny man. He had a competition going with a neighbor guy on who had the most lilac flowers on their bushes. F used to sneak up to my large lilac bush, cut flowers and tape them on his bush to win. I never knew. That was in March and Easter was coming up, so Den and I walked to meet each other on Easter Sunday, and then I walked back to the camp with him to meet some of his family. He was only staying there per doctor's orders, until he got his drain out and was able to get around on his own. He had a small house in Pownal.

Eventually, I became the love of his life. He brought me flowers, opened the car door to let me in, and opened it to let me out. He was always there for me. This talented and ambitious gentleman has treated me and my girls with love and care ever since. In the front room of our, then, farmhouse, he got on one knee, not the surgical knee, and asked me to marry him. I immediately said, yes. Den and I got married later that same year.

My girls and I welcomed J and S into our home. All the "kids" have always gotten along well. It was just meant to be. Den mostly worked from home, so it was an easy transition. They moved into the farmhouse, and everyone did fine. At least as fine as five teens can.

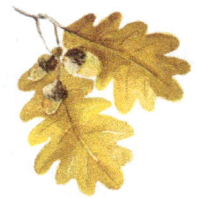

RAISING FIVE TEENS IS NOT, BY ANY MEANS, TROUBLE-FREE

Den never interfered in how I chose to discipline my girls, as I did not with his kids, (I did kick the steak knife, or was it a butter knife, away from he and J as they rolled on the barn floor) but we listened to each other, maybe gave our opinions or ideas and a few times had to both ride to the high school to retrieve the vehicle that one of them took to school when they were told not to. We managed a family trip to the Bahamas, Small Hope Bay Lodge which is a dive resort, the Florida keys, and other smaller trips here and there.

We were a great team. We still are, especially when it comes to the grand kids. They do, however, get away with a whole lot more.

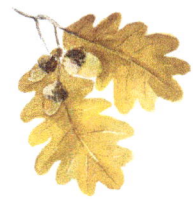

THE PRESSURE WAS RISING

I had been experiencing headaches for many years, increasing in intensity when I was pregnant. My headaches were getting worse, and the doctors would just say that I was "stressed," "I lost my husband," I was treated for sinus infections that I did not have, put on Xanax, a strong benzodiazepine, for neck tension "from stress," which "could be causing my headaches." Years later, it is still very difficult to get off this class of medication.

After 2 weeks of the worst headaches I had ever endured, continuously, I started seeing things floating in my peripheral vision. I also had vomited several times. My upset stomach was so bad one day, I had to leave work, call my PCP and insist I get an appointment I still had to wait a few days to get in but, it was finally time for a CT (computerized tomography) scan.

As I sat in the waiting room after the scan, wondering why I was sitting in the waiting room after the scan, the technician, who happened to be a friend from church, asked me and my husband, who for some reason, I had asked to come, to follow her to the telephone to speak to my PCP who had ordered the test. The light was shed on why I had such persistent headaches for the past ten years, and, to a lesser degree, still do. I had a colloid cyst blocking the cerebrospinal fluid from moving through the ventricles in my brain. I basically had been gradually increasing the amount of "water on my brain" over a lifetime. My head felt like a pressure cooker ready to explode.

Two years after getting re-married, I finally knew that the third ventricle was blocked causing hydrocephalus. My head still feels heavier than it should be, which is hard on my neck. I had brain surgery after taking Decadron for a week to decrease the swelling on my brain. Decadron is a strong steroid, and it did help me while I waited to have brain surgery.

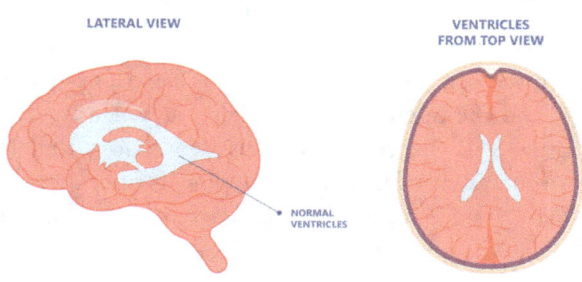

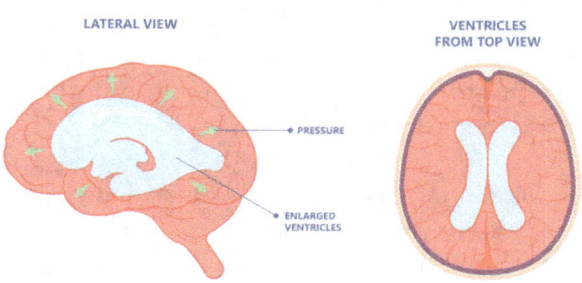

Brain ventricles

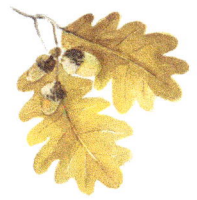

"YOU NEED BRAIN SURGERY, MORE SOONER, THAN LATER"

Here begins a list of some of the 30 plus practitioners that I received treatment from, over the years from 2009 to 2014 with 100% of two different "mesh kits" in my body. I include my brain surgeon first because down the "road of mesh," he is also the "beginning to my attempted finale," with this toxic, invasive, destructive material.

#1: Dr. B.

D r. K.B. MD is the exceptionally talented neurosurgeon who did my brain surgery on February 11 of 1999 in Portland, Maine. The day was memorable from that very early morning while my husband and I were sitting alone in that big waiting room and on the news, someone was reporting accusations of what sexual preference "Tinky Winky," the purple Teletubby, had. I sat there listening and then thinking it was kind of an odd thing to make it onto the news. A "Teletubby" is a stuffed animal? My husband was snoozing, so I am not 100% sure if this actually happened. At this point I started to think that maybe it was a good thing I was going to have brain surgery.

It was also my dad's birthday, so I thought of him as I was going under. From then on, every birthday of my dad's is now also called "*brain surgery day*."

The pre-anesthesia drugs that they gave me caused instant amnesia. Like the flip of a switch. Not surprisingly, I do not remember much right after the surgery. The first thing I remember was apparently about three days later, having a disturbing episode of "ICU (intensive care unit) psychosis." I woke up thinking I was tied in a chair and that people were trying to kill me. I was extremely paranoid, I was sure that I was being drugged through my intravenous line. I was sure someone, maybe my husband, was going to kill me. In my fury, I reached for my left hand, and I pulled out the IV catheter. This lessened the prospect of a quick return to lucidity, because there was now no quick, IV, access for drugs to be administered.

There were several people standing around me trying to orient me, including my husband, who I was hysterically afraid was going to reach into his pocket for lethal drugs and kill me. I remember saying that we had only been married for two years. *I still feel horrible about this.* I literally insisted that he empty his pockets onto the tray table, which he did. Finally, I noticed a pregnant nurse standing right beside me. Her ID tag had her first name and Maine Medical Center on it. For some reason seeing her, along with the intramuscular Haldol injection taking hold, I was finally able to settle down. Apparently, I was in my bed in the neuro ICU, not a chair. I am reminded from time to time that the first thing I said to one of my daughters was, "Don't ever let anyone mess with your brain." UGH, not fun!

It felt like days before I woke to my sweet neighbor, my angel, L or my husband Den. They were tag teaming, staying with me, or going home. I had a person with me all the time. I can truly say now that having them there made such a difference in my well-being. Looking back at what they both gave up and what they took on proves their commitment to me. It was a long ride into Portland twice a day to be by my side.

Twice, my urinary catheter bag was so full, it had backed all the way up into my bladder. I felt like my bladder would burst. I could hear the aide coming my way, the sound of metal and draining liquid. Whoever was with me got the aide to come quickly and empty it. I was looking for scissors or anything to cut the "balloon" line so I could pull that sucker out. I believe they were very short-staffed. If you are in the hospital, you should have someone with you.

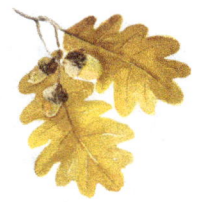

MORNING RITUALS

I do remember hearing the jingling of Dr. B's keys as he did his rounds in the neuro ICU very early most mornings. When he got to me, I could smell his cologne. *He reminded me of my late husband.* These morning rounds, most of which I can't remember in their entirety, were comforting to me. I had and still have full trust in Dr. B. He will be the, "beginning to the end," of my mesh catastrophe.

In the ICU, the head of my bed had to be kept at a certain level to match where the shunt was coming out of my brain. I do remember being in the upright position all the time. On another exceptionally unpleasant day, I remember having a headache that I could not bear. No number of drugs would decrease the intensity. Another CT (computerized topography) scan was ordered **STAT**. Even so, I remember being wheeled through a hallway, *it smelled of fear*, to eventually end up at the back of a very long line of wheelchairs and stretchers. I remember a great feeling of doom.

I am not sure how long I waited. My husband was with me. The next thing I remember was being back in the neuro ICU and Dr. B's PA (physician's assistant) saying, the CT scan was unchanged and "pull the shunt." Once they pulled the shunt tube from my brain, I had instant relief and was transferred the next day to the regular neuro floor and promptly forgotten.

I was in a room with an unresponsive roommate. I could not get anyone to help me up to the commode after being in bed for 8 days. I gladly took the inflation devices off my legs. I had contemplated taking a sharp instrument to these as well. They are necessary to prevent clot formation and a potential traveling clot that can land in your lungs or your heart or your brain. But *I was getting up* so I didn't need those irritating, lifesaving balloon pumps anymore. I had to get to the commode, thankfully, only about four feet away, by myself. I had told Den to go home for some much-needed rest and he did, because I called home, a landline, still no cell phones, and got the answering machine. I couldn't believe no one on my nursing floor was answering my call light. I managed to somehow get myself to the commode. Someone did finally come to answer my call and I requested a popsicle, which I never got. Again, short staffed.

I didn't realize it at the time but there was a possibility that I would go home with a permanent shunt that would drain excess fluid off my brain and into my chest or abdominal cavity. This shunt from the ventricle in my brain would have been tunneled under the skin along the side of my head and neck into the chosen cavity (chest or abdominal) to be reabsorbed by my body. Twenty-five years later, now, my skull is still tender at the operative sites. My body doesn't seem to like foreign substances in it anywhere.

At 12 weeks post brain surgery, I went back to work part time, took care of my family to the best of my ability, continued taking my RN to BSN classes, and now I had a reason for the "elevens," age lines between my eyebrows, which had been present for several years due to the chronic headaches. But I want to stress that even with all that, I returned to work! I was never one to wallow in things or lay down and quit. I did hang on to that branch at the edge of the Live Oak tree.

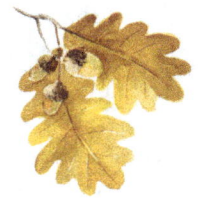

GET YOUR PAP SMEARS &
MAMMOGRAMS LADIES

#2: Dr. W, MD, gynecology

Dr. W is an MD in Maine. She has been my gynecologist for 20 years. In the winter of 2008-2009, I saw Dr. W because of the heavy bleeding and cramping I was experiencing along with being in the menopausal age group. She is a great doctor with a wonderful bedside manner. She always showed interest in my complete healthy state of being. Because we were going to move to Florida, I did not pursue the possibility of having surgery in Maine with her. Oh man, how I wish I had. Maybe things would have turned out differently.

I trusted Dr. W and she told me I was suffering from Adenomyosis. This is a condition in which extra cells that usually line the uterus (endometrium, see pic) were instead inside my uterine walls. Each month, as hormones dictated, my entire uterus, the walls included, were engorged with blood causing cramping and heavy bleeding.

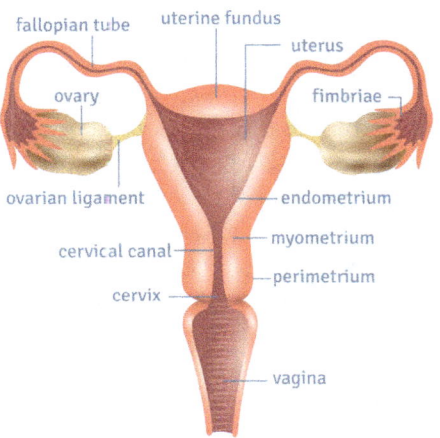

Female reproductive system

Also, perhaps mostly because of chronic constipation, due likely to pain medication, I had also started to "prolapse" most of my pelvic organs. By the time I had surgery in 2009, my bladder had prolapsed to a stage one. This was not so bad and I had no urinary incontinence at this point. My uterus, however, had shifted down blocking my vagina and laying onto my rectum. This was a third degree prolapse and not good. I was able to temporarily manage things myself until we got to Florida, where I got a second opinion. I would eventually need a hysterectomy and prolapse repairs. My husband was returning from Iraq and I was working in a job that I would not abandon due to the personal and finite nature of it. I felt I could wait until we got to Florida.

Most specialists will only treat problems related to their specialty. Over those worst five years of my life, living in that live oak tree, meeting dead end after dead end, while the plastic mesh silently invaded all areas of my pelvic cavity, I saw so many practitioners, not just MD's but pain specialists, neurosurgeons, chiropractors, seven different physical therapists, to name only some. They all seemed convinced that my pain was coming from a potential or old spinal disc injury, or complications of an injury.

Although I knew that most acute disc injuries caused pain down at least one leg by way of the sciatic nerve, I kept seeking the answer. All I could really do was rule out the "injury to my disc" theory that had been continually thrown in my face. Being so, when I flew north in 2014, at my wits' end, I did not even go see Dr. W because at this point, I knew to my core, that it was the mesh causing me to feel so debilitated and unable to function as a woman of my age should. Pain from a herniated disc does not last for five years, nor does it cause a person to feel as if they are being poisoned. I am continuing my yearly checks with her now. She prescribes hormone therapy for me.

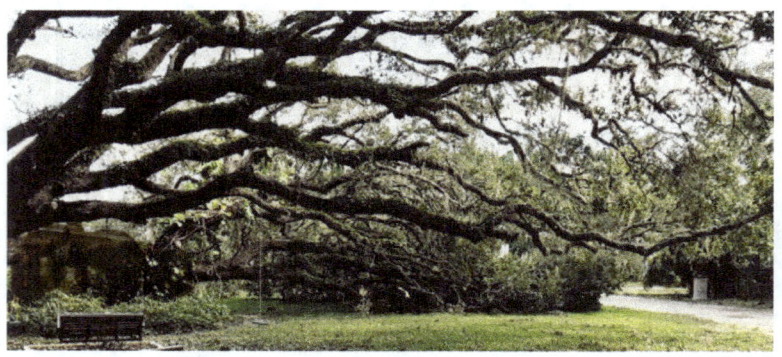

My live oak tree

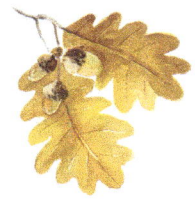

ALWAYS THERE FOR ME

#3: Dr. B, MD, Primary Care Provider 2008-2019, Saint Augustine, Florida

I found Dr. B after I joined my husband in Florida. She was a kind and gentle woman. Den went to Saint Augustine ahead of me for his work commitment and to start the process of finding us a house. I stayed back and prepared to sell our house in Maine.

Unfortunately, we were forced to put it up for rent. We had two undesirable tenants. The first family was by far the worst. They did not communicate with our management company, and they stopped paying their rent with no explanation or willingness to work things out.

Renting out property can be a real challenge unless you get lucky with a good management company, which is needed if you live far away from the rental property. Finding understanding, considerate tenants is a process that our managers did not go through. We had hired one of the two rental management companies advertised in our area not realizing that we were their first customers.

We asked them to start the eviction process and they did go to court on our behalf. Police were sent to the house to escort the tenants out, but of course, there were kids involved so the state of Maine was not going to throw a family out on the streets. When the eviction was complete, the tenants had caused considerable damage to the house and left the garage full of trash. They were also growing marijuana in the basement in a time when it was illegal. Dark hair dye stained the kitchen floor and the old wood window sills of this beautiful Victorian home.

Our second tenants, unbeknownst to us, had a connection to our management, husband/wife team. Their daughters went to school together. These folks treated our house with more care and respect but were only able to pay their rent through the husband doing projects around the house that he deemed necessary. We finally sold the home and took a significant loss.

These years around (2007-2009) were, financially, tough for a lot of people. My husband rented a condominium in Saint Augustine, temporarily, while looking at houses and working from home. We decided we wanted to live near the beach, which had always been a dream for me. This dream came true while we were under contract on a house five blocks from the beach. I did not like the house or the "Stepford wife" look of the neighborhood at all but felt we had run out of options.

We were just about to close on this obnoxious excuse for a house, when the bank claimed that there was a $90,000 lien on this property. Just at this time, our Realtor knew of a young couple who were struggling financially and thinking of selling their beautiful bungalow surrounded by live oaks and just a half block from the Matanzas River. Luckily, it was in the same development of the other home, just a few blocks farther from the beach still on Anastasia Island. We bought this house instead. Being close to the beach really was a big part of getting me through the worst ten years of my life. I just wish I could have enjoyed it more.

Dr. B, my PCP, was part of a healthcare system affiliated with a hospital in Jacksonville. In the beginning, the visits were short as most doctor visits are today. This was especially stressful on me after my mesh implant because I felt like I was being poisoned and my low back pain and instability was getting worse every day. Every appointment, and there were so many, was torture. Dr. B and I became "professional" friends, and we shared family stories and photos of our families. I followed Dr. B to a practice she shared with one other doctor and then to her own practice that was a pay by the month system with patients having access to Dr. B or a covering doctor, whenever needed. At least that was the goal, and the visits I experienced met my expectations. I know Dr. B believed that I was in pain. I also believe that she didn't know why. I could count on her, my one "rock" in a "sea of kelp."

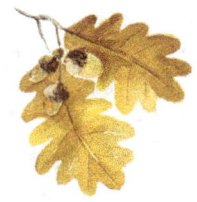

HERE I AM AGAIN

#4: K, NP, gynecology, worked with Dr. B

My visits to Dr. B's, NP, K were quite frequent and a long distance from my home. K had a particular interest in women's health. Many physicians pair up with nurse practitioners, who see patients in their practice, and I believe K got a bit tired of seeing me. She was who I saw most often. When I was there for complaints concerning urinary issues, my visits were very frequent and short. I was uncomfortable all the time.

The female anatomy is the perfect setup for bacteria to travel the short distance from the rectal opening (anus) where E. coli bacteria normally exists, to the urethral opening, where E. coli most frequently causes urinary tract infections in women. There are many ladies, young and old, who do not realize that they have three "openings" in their perineum. This is why, when I worked with patients in various settings, I always taught them about their anatomy and the importance of great hygiene. I had more than one lady tell me she thought she "peed out of her vagina." I impressed on them the importance of wiping from front to back, after a bowel movement, to help avoid contamination and a potential urinary tract infection.

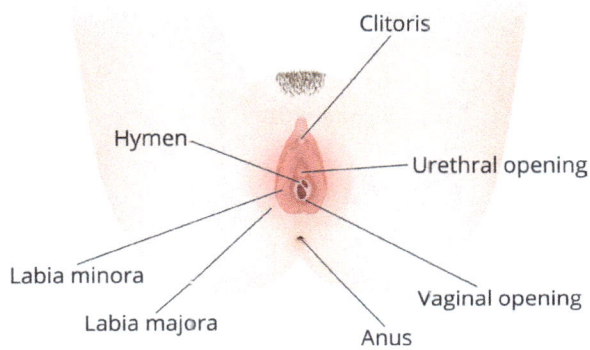

Three orifices of the female perineum are shown above: urethral opening, vaginal opening and anus.

K decided that sex was causing my problems, although at this time, mini sling implanted, sexual activity for me was uncomfortable. I was working with pelvic floor physical therapists to try to improve my intimacy. She prescribed Macrobid, an antibiotic to be taken after every sexual encounter. Taking antibiotics routinely was extremely detrimental for my gut health and led to other problems like chronic vaginal yeast infections. She neglected to add probiotics to my health regimen.

I am sure that many of the women reading this book can relate to this. The problem was not my hygiene. It was the mini-sling mesh, that at that time I did not know was now implanted in my vaginal wall. It was like two open sores, one on each side of my vagina, as well as the irritation of the mesh inside the wall of tissue.

I so wish I had asked more questions around my hysterectomy surgery. Who equates mesh in the vaginal wall with a hysterectomy? I believe my surgeon felt he was doing me a favor. It was 2009 when the mesh went in and the controversy of mesh had just begun being investigated in the U.S. in 2008, although, I am seeing now on social media that women were having problems way before then.

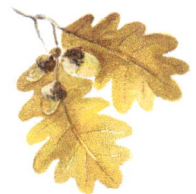

IMPLANTED MESH IN 2009 & REMOVED ALL HE COULD IN 2014

#5: Dr. M in Atlanta, GA, offered surgery to do a hysterectomy with removal of the complete uterus, and given my age, 50 years old at that time, removing both ovaries. This would eliminate the chance of ovarian cancer, which is prevalent after the menopausal years. He would also fix all prolapses. This could all be done by laparoscopy with "very small incisions and a quick recovery." This doctor is world renowned for helping women all over the world with many unusual gynecologic problems. I do not believe he meant me any harm.

I met Dr. M. in August of 2009. He explained the surgery, showed me a soft piece of 2" x 2" mesh, and he drew the diagram pictured below. This attempted to compare my anatomy to what a normal woman would be. His explanation of the surgery did not make me connect this small piece of mesh to the prolapse repair.

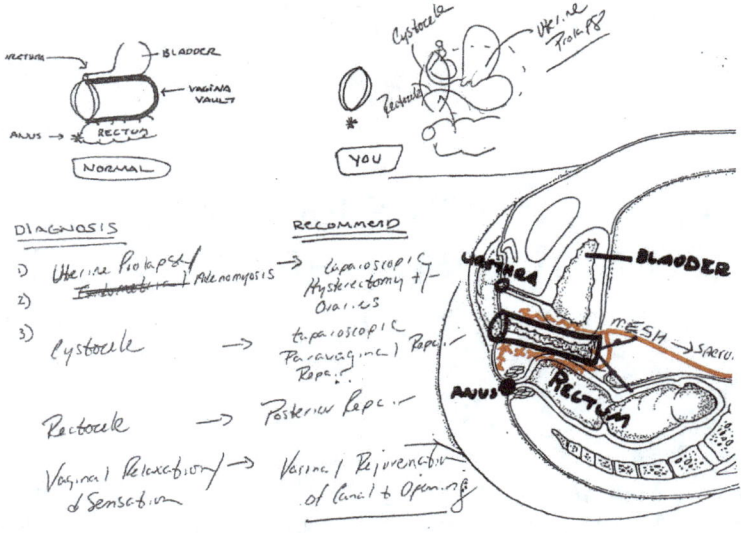

Showing normal perineal anatomy in upper left (lateral view) and what my anatomy looked like in upper right. The larger diagram attempted to show placement of the much bigger sacral coccygeal Y mesh which was placed following the removal of my uterus (hysterectomy). I did not understand the diagram until later when I researched the surgery and added the red color to show the mesh placement from the vaginal walls to the sacrum or tailbone, marked by an arrow pointing backwards.

My surgery was scheduled for Sept 29, 2009. I added to his diagram in red to show the sacral coccygeal Y mesh in red wrapped around the vaginal walls and being attached to the sacrum where I put an arrow. This pulling on my sacrum was felt by me within one month of mesh implantation. The pulling caused my pelvic fragility and instability that is only known to the person who is experiencing it. It was terrifying to feel like I was a puppet on a string that could break at any moment, and I didn't know why.

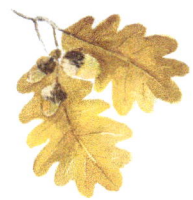

VAMPIRE BABY

Waking up from this surgery felt like I had "the vampire baby from hell" in my pelvis. *I had just read the Twilight series*, which is not my usual genre, but, suggested and borrowed from my daughter. I had read so many books and watched so many series, that I got hooked.

If you are not familiar with this supposed "teenage series," at the end, the human girl is pregnant with her vampire lover's baby. My whole abdomen felt like something was inside of me fighting "tooth and nail" to get out. There was no making me comfortable and, like always, staffing was low. My nurse tried, I will give her that, but it was most likely all the gas they injected into my pelvic cavity to allow them to laparoscopically see all my organs easier. Doing things, the easier way is not AT ALL always the best way.

Laparoscopic surgery was the new thing, and the mesh made the procedure easier for the surgeon. Easier means quicker, quicker means more surgeries, more surgeries mean more money. At least that is how I see it now.

After returning to the operating room that evening because of uncontrolled bleeding from my vagina, I had the memory of someone pushing on my throat, like trying to choke me. I know as a nurse that if a patient must return to surgery and has had anything to drink, even water, they apply pressure to the larynx to prevent aspiration during tube placement. But at that moment, all I knew was pain in my throat. I yelled and jerked awake, and the anesthesia person promptly gave me more medications. I was out again; I honestly don't remember much more about my hospital stay other than trying to urinate so I could be discharged. That never happened in the hospital.

I honestly don't remember much more than trying to urinate so I could be discharged. That never happened in the hospital, and I was sent home to self-catheterize my urine until I was healed. Why didn't I question this development?

I am Woman, Hear me Roar.
—HELEN REDDY

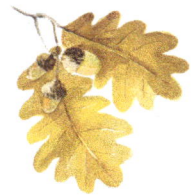

A NEVER-ENDING RECOVERY

For me, and most likely most implant recipients, the V shaped part of the Y mesh, placed upside down holding the vagina on each side, from inside the pelvic cavity, was irritating and working its way inside the vaginal walls. Many women become aware that the mesh is eroding into their vagina by their sexual partner who can sometimes feel a scratching or scraping pain during intercourse.

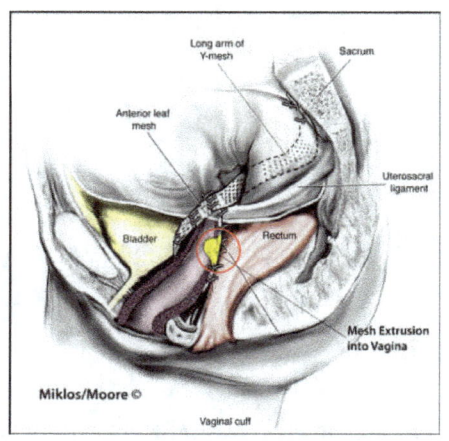

Picture of mesh eroding into vagina.

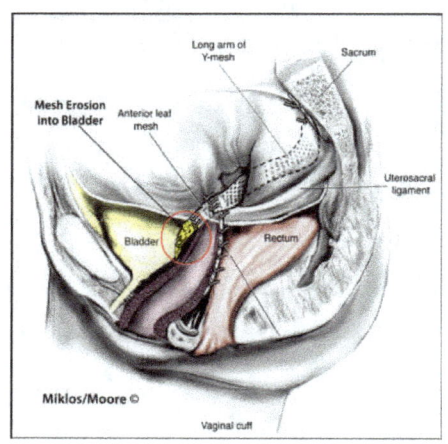

Picture of mesh eroding bladder.

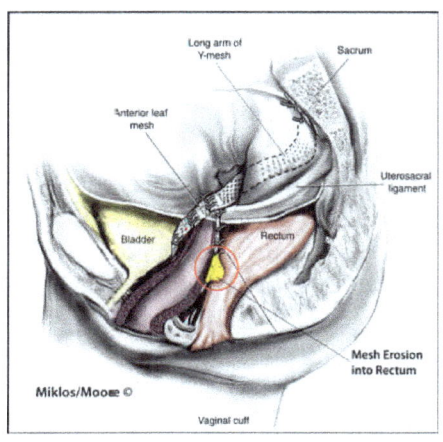

Picture of mesh eroding bowel.

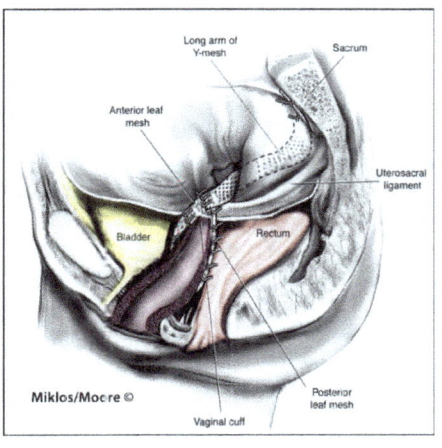

Picture of mesh sewn in with no erosion.

This being the sacrococcygeal mesh, the other tail end of the Y shaped mesh (again upside-down Y) was sewn into my sacrum, or tailbone, causing a pulling sensation as it crimped and shrunk causing my pelvic pain, extreme low back pain, a fragile feeling of instability, and bilateral hip pain. These symptoms for me, started about a month after the surgery.

The generalized feeling of being poisoned grew increasingly worse over the five years that the mesh was inside my body. There seemed to be a gradual increase in nausea which no doctors cared to investigate. Most of the woman on the support groups on social media sites confirm having this feeling of being poisoned. My PCP prescribed Zofran for me to help lessen the nausea. I did read online that many mesh products are treated with certain chemicals. I have also read accounts from woman and men online, stating that the mesh they obtain from areas it erodes to are many different colors. This indicated to me that perhaps dyes are used. I was really starting to lose it by this point.

The second mesh, the "mini-sling," "*the bonus,*" was burrowed into the walls of the vaginal opening placed in such a way to support the urethra, the tube from the bladder to the outside of the body. Many women have only this mesh in them. A cure for their incontinence. But the tragedies from this piece of small plastic migrating into their bladder, cutting their urethra's in half, destroying their ability to urinate normally, completely ruining their lives, are many. This I know from the various online social media groups.

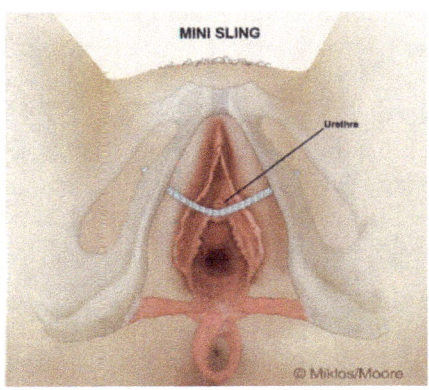

Mesh is pushed into vaginal walls and hung under urethra to help with urinary incontinence.

For me, the urinary issues were uncomfortable and misleading, causing me to take urinary pain pills almost continuously. I blamed those symptoms on life as well as all the catheters I used post op. I blamed it on having three babies, being menopausal and any other issue that we women may face. I curse myself every day for not knowing that Dr. M implanted two mesh devices during that surgery. I still take urinary pain pills for several days in a row every so often, I live as if I have a constant UTI. I only wear cotton underwear and of course a leakage pad every day, I wear mostly pull-on stretchy pants, drink a lot of water, pee a lot, and take Uribel.

But at that time, my mind was so focused on my lower back and pelvis being painful and unstable, that I dreaded waking up every morning, which is still the worst time of day for me. My life is dictated by getting through the activities of daily living. My husband has been doing the grocery shopping and cooking. I am gradually getting back into walking with the "silver sneakers" program. It allows me to do only what I can do.

Certain activities are still painful. I'm guessing this is because, like my neck, muscles have memory. I watch every step I take, especially on cobblestones, uneven ground, as well as on the beach, boardwalks, docks, and anywhere there is a dip in the pavement. Bending just a little is still painful, as is lifting, pushing, and pulling. This is what was wreaking havoc on my everyday life and thankfully has improved quite a bit. I do however, still love when my family thinks to hold on to me if we are walking in the dark.

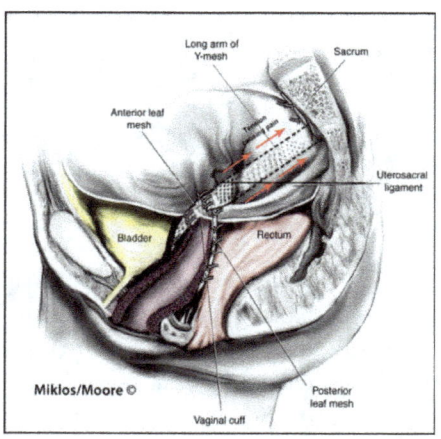

The mesh is pulling causing vaginal pain. IN my case the majority of my pain was from the pulling on my sacrum (low back) and my vagina as shown in diagram This diagram does not show any erosion It is pushed Into the vaginal walls and "hung" under the urethra to help with urinary incontinence.

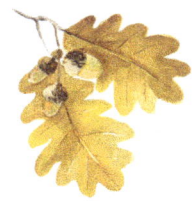

I LIVED IN MY LIVE OAK TREE EVERY DAY, GAZING FROM BED.

Pain is Subjective, and I Am Broken

One day, as I remember it, I was sitting on my bed in St. Augustine, Florida, tearful, and full of hopelessness. I have been on several different antidepressants over the years as well as having seen at least five different therapists. I look at depression as a silent killer. Kind of like high blood pressure, it must be known and then treated.

Watching the squirrels run through the highway of branches sprawling from the trunk of my lovely, centuries-old, live Oak tree, I pictured myself barely hanging on to the most outer point of the branches. The Spanish moss brushing by whispering for me to let go, I saw myself as weak and small, hanging there, running out of strength, not knowing whether to let go or take a deep breath and pull myself up.

I am broken! I can still see myself there. Am I crazy? I had been to so many places, seen so many different practitioners, eastern and western medicine, and yet, there I was, hanging from the branch alone, sick, and scared. The suffering is unbearable. No one else knows how I feel.

Every time I try to head to the stronger part of the tree, where stability could be, where I could find answers and relief, I run into dead ends. My head hurts so much from slamming into torment. I am trying desperately to get on the branch to health. No matter which way I go, I must turn around and retreat. No one can help me. I have survived so many traumas in my life.

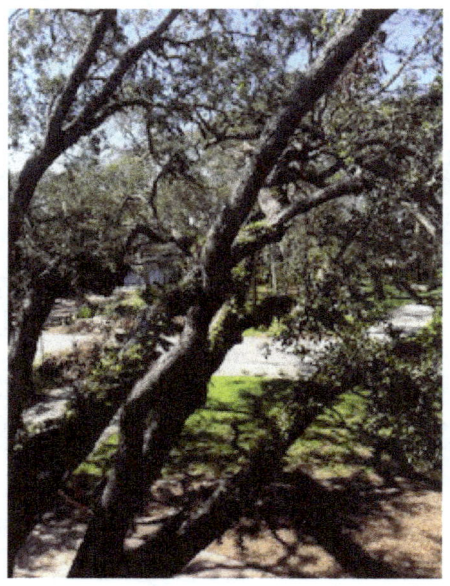

Live oak tree

There must be an answer and maybe it is the answer to the question that I asked Dr. M, my surgeon, one month after he implanted that foreign mesh inside my pelvis. "Could the mesh be causing my new onset back pain?" Back then he said, "Absolutely no! Less than one percent of women have any trouble." Things change, especially inside the human body. I will not give up. I was running circles in the live oak tree, still hitting the dead ends hard with no one there to catch me.

Compassion fatigue is a real issue. I can certainly understand why my family and friends would start to "not hear my complaints." I think I, too, had compassion fatigue. I was tired of complaining I was losing hope. But I could not and would not live my life under these circumstances. NO WAY! I needed to find my trail back to myself. Back to the trunk and roots of the live oak that stood for so long."

Thankfully, my husband worked from home. He took good care of me, and he never doubted my pain. I do not, however, believe that he understood the gravity of my situation. Why would he? I am the nurse. Even so, my family was my magnet. It was their pull that I felt when times were the worst.

I wobbled around on the edge of life's ridges, challenging many people who were "experts" in their field, complying through such pain by baring teeth and getting it done. I exposed my body to unknown drugs. Many injections, painful maneuvers, and more! But not once did I fall all the way off that ledge to the abyss. I grabbed for everything that was in front of me. Acupuncture, Reiki, massage, essential oils, "healing waters," and any other things that was suggested, plus all the conventional approaches I had already tried. I took a chance on myself. I needed answers.

I mustered up the strength and pulled myself up and continued asking for help. I did not quit. I was so tired of being told that my weak core was the problem even after I had been doing Pilates twice a week for two and half years. From the very beginning I have been a compliant patient. That is the reason I did not qualify for disability on three occasions. The lawyer I was working with was only seeking back payment for the worst two years. But because I did what I was told. I "walked on the beach." The judge denied me every time.

best Mommy in the World!

so thankful for your
love and judge-free
No matter what I know
there for me and I
on you. Thank you
at. I love you so so
I feel spoiled to have you
mum!
you soon,
XOXO
am me because of

build
pe of loving
at I come

Uni

love and app
ou and all yo
For us, big a

the best momma eva!
Thank you for being you
raising me to be stro
hank you for thriving
he hardest times of
hat has always and
you conquer challe
our faith in God ha
eatest example to u
m forever grateful.
w/ all n

You're non-judgemental prospective and unconditional love mean the world to

I want you
ow that it come
the strongest love
ever. Mother +
ter love
You mea
e wide world to me.
Love you so much

ive up being there for me and
demonstrating kindness, love
and compassion. I learned that
from you and its helped me
every day. I love you
for always
for all
elp. Y
st M
e wid

Lov

I'm proud of your persistence
ve I truly love you to the moon
very much with + more.
all my heart! hope to pay
kindness for

dn't be where I am
ithout you blessings Love you so

'Life doesn't come with a manual, it comes with a mother! Thank you for all you do for us. Hope you have a relaxing day! Love

with all my ...

... my lucky stars ...day that you ...my mom. The ...things in life ...to do with you ...d our family ...nd the legacy we have built together and for our sweet next generation. Sweet babies Cale + Sage. Thank you! Love you forever.

Thank God that we ... so close ...dn't even be... to thank you enough. You been so great to me an... supporting. You are so sm... beautiful, loving, caring a... fun. I'm so proud to have you as my Mom.
I love you

Thank you mom... for always being you. We are so lucky to have such a beautiful, thoughtful, smart and loving mother. Thanks for making us us! Happy Valentine's Da...

...have to say that ...re not an easy mom to
Without I value your ...on so much.

...est Nana ever

...a unicorn! I could... you real... for a better mother, friend, confidan... system. You are always there for...

Love you so

...erish every ...for every ...

Thank you so much for all ...and support.

Love you so

...u have done ...d always L ...when we n ...most!

Momma,
.I love and respect ...

So proud of you for doing... It just proves you can do...

I love my ...so much and I look... you and value your o... and insights more th...

Imagine

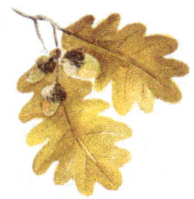

BRAINWAVES

#6: Dr. G., MD, Naturopath

This doctor used unconventional methods to *try to* help his patients. Most people would consider him handsome and quite debonair. He was a good listener and he seemed to care.

He immediately recommended his own physical therapist to me. Most of his emphasis was using Asyra testing. On his webpage it says this testing is a non-invasive, quick way to evaluate factors related to your health. I thought it might pinpoint areas in the body that were not in sync. Each visit, I held two metal handles which fed information to a machine.

I saw Dr. G for several months. I was no better. I convinced my husband to go try the Asyra machine. When we left the office, my husband said, "That is a crock of shit." I must say that I agree since there was plastic mesh invading my entire pelvic cavity and his "machine" did not detect it. He suggested the use of some over the counter herbs and teas.

I ended our appointments when 1.) the office refused to accommo-
date my request to change my appointments to the town I lived in—I
was not told he even had a satellite office—and 2.) he made me feel
uncomfortable by sharing personal information that I considered
unprofessional. I got no guidance or relief from Dr. G. He was an
internal medicine MD but did not seem to concentrate on what was
inside my body at all.

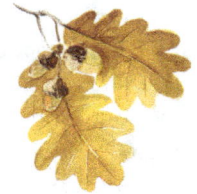

WE ARE WHAT WE EAT

#7: Dr. K, acupuncture

D r. K was highly recommended and said to be the best acupuncturist in the area. He was a nice guy who listened to my concerns, but after no relief of my low back pain from the acupuncture, he could only offer food allergy testing which showed that I had one genetic marker for celiac disease, which my sister has, and that I had a yeast infection "throughout my entire body." He did not offer medications, just a yeast free diet. You would be surprised how many foods have yeast in them. I have found more recently that if I have signs of a yeast infection, especially after antibiotics, taking probiotics has given me the best results. No help from Dr. K.

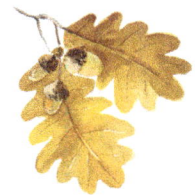

STEP OUTSIDE THE BOX

#8: PM, NP

I saw a women's health specialist for three months. She had previously worked with a doctor who wrote a popular book on women's health, so I was hopeful I might get some answers. I was experiencing continuous vaginal and urinary tract infections.

As before, nothing unusual showed up in my vaginal culture or urinalysis. She was not the warm and fuzzy type, but their office took my insurance, so I decided it was worth a try. It turned out to be a waste of time and gas money. She talked me into purchasing expensive supplements. She also ordered and pretty much insisted that I have more lab tests for Lyme disease and food allergies, which insurance did not cover. I was desperate!

She monitored my progress every other week but at the end of the summer nothing had changed. Like most of the providers her face kind of glazed over when I suggested my back pain might be from the Y mesh in my pelvis. She was not interested enough to request records from my implant surgery. If she had, things could have been much better for me. As it was, I got no help from her either.

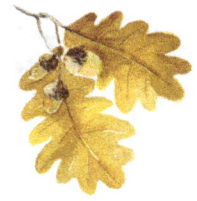

SCHEDULE MY LIFE

During these times of going from appointment to appointment, I would try to schedule as many rest days as possible. At the beginning of every day, I dreaded waking up because I knew that I would be in debilitating pain.

I lived my life in slow motion, planning every move, watching every step, everywhere I went, every day, and by the end of every day, in which I did any physical activity at all, I literally could not get into my house without help. It always happened, that once I sat for a while, in my car or in a chair, and then prepared to get up, I could not walk without help. Now, I can understand why. This still happens rarely if I overdo it physically. *The more I do, the more I hurt.*

Prior to the mesh removal surgery, my bed, with either heat or ice, was always my destination. Now I have a favorite comfy chair and thankfully the episodes of debilitating spams are occurring much less often. I also had to keep up with the routine appointments that come around yearly for myself, and for my disabled sister-in-law. I am, after all, a nurse. I did want to make sure she was getting good care especially because I was not. Both she and my husband's alcoholic brother followed us to Florida, and I tried to help the best I could with both.

We received help from our youngest daughter and her husband during the hurricanes. They were living in Florida and still are. With our other children spread out in the country, I was on my own a lot and I was often the one doing the nurturing. The autoimmune issues, particularly the 'Hashimoto's Thyroiditis," lessened my appetite. This also further decreased my will to move my body. I was retaining water and gaining weight.

I could not have survived these years without my husband. I was feeling like I had tried everything. I'm sure that most of the practitioners that I saw were thinking I was a hypochondriac or possibly seeking drugs. I only ever realized that this mindset would occur, when I quickly discarded and reported Dr. C, who was a "pain specialist," or that is what he referred to himself as.

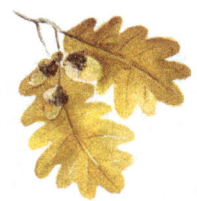

"LETTERS TO A YOUNG POET"

A Poem by Rainer Maria Rilke

.... have patience in everything that remains unsolved in your heart, try to love the questions themselves, like locked rooms and like books written in a foreign language. Do not now look for the answers. They can not now be given to you, because you could not live them. It is a question of experiencing everything. At present you need to live the question. Perhaps you will gradually. Without even noticing it, find yourself experiencing the answer. Some distant day.

I think there are a lot of ways to interpret this poem. I certainly did need patience and strength to hold on to the "limb" of that live oak. The answer would come, with persistence and self-confidence, as it did with my headaches. It is unfortunate it had to take so long. I feel so angry and sad for the thousands or perhaps millions of women who are suffering still and not knowing why. I pray this book will help many.

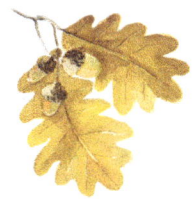

SHOULD COMPLIANCE BE PUNISHED?

#9: Dr. P, MD, Cardiology

I was seeing Dr. P on a regular basis because I have had and still have a resting heart rate of over 100 beats per minute, which accelerates quickly up to 120 with mild activity. I had many tests, including a stress test and an echocardiogram, which were normal other than the initial resting heart rate of 116. It did not take long for my heart rate to reach the level they wanted it to reach.

After a second opinion, it was decided that my tachycardia must be a result of my chronic pain. Dr. P, especially, wanted me to pay attention to my heart health. He wanted me to walk at least twice a week. Dr. P documented this in my record, which is the only record the judge talked about during my disability hearings. I was not allowed time to say what I had prepared.

This second in-person hearing was on a holiday weekend and late on a Friday. The hearing ended quickly. It seemed in this judge's eyes, if a person is disabled, they must just lie in bed all day. My lawyer did his best, but I guess I was just *too much of* a compliant patient. The fact that I walked on the beach is what, yet again, denied me compensation for what is owed to me *from the work that I would have loved to continue.*

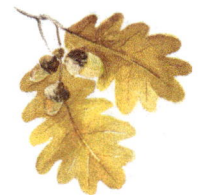

"OVER THE BRIDGE, INTO THE LION'S MOUTH"

#10: Dr. T, Psychologist, PhD

With the pain and nausea that I experienced every minute of every day, I felt like I was falling deeper and deeper into a black hole. I believe I saw at least seven therapists/psychologists for my depression and for the impending feeling of doom that I could not shake.

My husband attended one session with me. I could not sit and try to make Dr. T and my husband understand what I was going through. At this appointment I got so upset I ran out of the office, *in the worst shoes possible, of course*, and headed to downtown Saint Augustine toward the "Bridge of Lions." I was determined that I would walk the six miles home.

I needed to be by myself for a while because my life was spinning out of control. I kept thinking of the chance of this being a permanent physical and mental state of health for me, worsening with each day until I would *finally* die. People, including doctors, were tired of hearing my story of chronic pain and now I was at the end point. It had to be the mesh.

My husband found me on the other side of the bridge, sitting on the ground against a brick wall. The tears finally came. How can a therapist or a husband help a person who is in pain because they have been wronged surgically, and don't even know it?

Please look around at your loved ones. Have they had surgery? Are they feeling well? Are they incontinent? I shudder to think of how many women are going through what I went through, which was at this time at an extremely high level of so many things all jumbled together.

Now, I am trying to improve self-care and move ahead the best I can, hopefully helping women and/or men become aware that this problem is or could become a horrible epidemic. One with no vaccine or cure. Please say no to mesh.

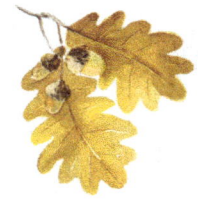

THE SHOCK OF MY LIFE

#11: Dr. C, DO, Pain Management

I decided that I needed to go to a doctor who specialized in pain control. Looking online, I found Dr. C, who was not too far from my house. At my first visit, and from the moment I locked eyes with this man, I could sense a feeling of adverse judgment from him. He spoke very little to me and in a condescending way. I felt like he had already decided that I was guilty of something, until proven innocent. This created an unsettled feeling inside me.

Without any introduction or giving me any chance to tell him my history, he told me I would have to take a "drug profile" lab test. This was *not* covered by insurance, and he wanted the money upfront. That man tested me for every legal and illegal medication that existed. He checked for cocaine, heroin, and for all the opioids, alcohol and many more. I am not sure if he wanted to confirm that I was taking my medications as prescribed? That would make sense and perhaps rule out that I was selling drugs.

He did not talk to me or explain any of the treatments. But just continued his pursuit of whatever crazy goal he had, like a robot. Why I did not turn around and leave right then, I am not sure.

In my desperation, I returned for my second visit in which he was apparently satisfied with my lab results, and so, he did a very quick exam of my reflexes and asked me to walk and bend. He told me that I needed a cortisone shot for a herniated disc and that I should schedule it on my way out. I explained that I had been a nurse for a long time and had no symptoms of sciatica. He did not say anything.

On my next and final visit, they brought me in a back room and had me lie down on a hard cold slab. *Maybe x-ray guided?* I thought. But I was soon sure that was not the case. There was another person there but no one explained anything. Before I even realized what he was doing, he pierced my low back with what felt like a very large needle, sending an excruciating bolt of electricity down my leg! He used no anesthetic. He gave no warning. The shock wave was unimaginable! I am pretty sure that I screamed and pushed myself up the best I could to a seated position. That was it! This "doctor" was cruel and who I would consider a "quack."

Once I was able to walk, I said nothing, I was shaking in fear and pain. I answered no questions, paid no money, and slowly got the hell out of that torture chamber. I reported this brute to the American Medical Association and hand-delivered a copy of the complaint to his office. On the way out, I met a woman going in and I told her she should "think twice." There was nothing at all positive about this doctor. I now realized that I had not only been stripped of my dignity, but I was also deeper in despair. Oh God, how long can this nightmare go on?

I decided I had to let it go. Let go of yet another traumatic experience. I had been invited to a Pampered Chef party and decided to give it a try. My life had been a series of scheduled appointments followed by so much discomfort that all I wanted was to stop! During the Pampered Chef party, I decided I would try becoming a Pampered Chef consultant. It felt nice to hang out with other women.

It was obvious to everyone that I walked very gingerly. I tried not to go into details but rather just let people know that I moved slow because of back issues. I totally didn't realize what I was getting into. I had to lug bags of cookware. Duh! I remember quite vividly at my first and only home show, sitting on a very uncomfortable stool, taking people's orders. I was so thirsty, and people were in a hurry. I was unable to move from the stool. Once everyone was gone, I asked the hostess's husband to carry my bags back to my car.

From then on, I did catalog shows only. I stayed with it for quite a while because the products were delivered right to the customers, so no heavy lifting for me. Once my family and friends had all they needed from Pampered Chef, I stopped being a consultant. Financially, I came out even, but all our kitchens are well-stocked with products I mostly love. At least I tried and the social interaction, even over the phone, made me feel more alive.

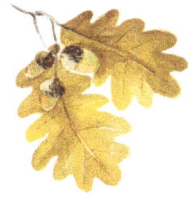

AM I LOSING IT?

What a conundrum for me and many other women who have and are still suffering the effects of surgical mesh. I was absolutely thinking I was going out of my mind. One of the many social media sites I found to support victims of mesh complications has over 10,000 members.

I know that other women are suffering far worse than I am. Had I not persisted in my quest to find out what was causing my symptoms, I too would be far worse off or perhaps dead. The mesh was attached to my bowel. Had it perforated the bowel wall and allowed excrement to spill into my peritoneal cavity, I could have become septic and died.

Sometimes being stoic isn't the best answer, especially in the case of women who are built to endure physical pain. We tend to be too sturdy sometimes causing us to ignore pain or unusual symptoms occurring in us. Don't suffer in silence, there is help available now and a whole new mindset on the use of mesh.

The guilt I feel is solidly placed in my mind and will be there forever. This is because I allowed a doctor to decide what was best for my body. I didn't do the research. I didn't read between the lines.

Again, I started to wonder if I was having serious psychiatric problems? Did my brain surgery mess up my pain tolerance? Why were none of the many treatments helping my pain and instability? My husband and I are approaching our retirement years. We had a plan which we are now struggling to attain because *I still do everything in* "*s l o w m o t i o n*" and by 2pm, I need to rest with heat or ice and pain medications. My life is forever changed.

I was supposed to be employed in a beautiful historical college in the "oldest city" in our country. I became a Nana on May the fourth ("*be with you*") in 2013! I am a wife, but not a very good one! My husband was picking up my slack. But now our lives are so full and complicated that it is too much even for him to help me.

I had worked either part time or full time for 30 years. My income was part of our future. As you can imagine, going to eastern medicine providers and having acupuncture, reflexology, massages, reiki, polarity and probably a couple more, the bills were expensive and not covered at all by insurance.

We were planning that my part-time job at the student health center was going to eventually turn into a full-time management position, since the current manager was to become a nurse practitioner, and I would be able to fall into her position. I really enjoyed being on campus with the college students and having a lot of acute care experience, the job was perfect. Unable to run to a student one day who had fallen down the stairs made me realize that I could no longer deny these young adults the quick reaction time they may need. The student was okay. I was very disappointed in myself.

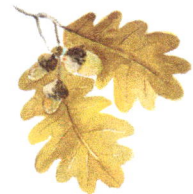

MINE & HIS = OURS

We have five adult children, who were, during our ten years living in Florida, very busy having babies, coming and going to Iraq, experiencing life trauma, on helicopter missions in Afghanistan, looking for jobs, running to bomb shelters in Bahram, getting married, graduating and so many other life events. There was so much that I wanted to be involved in.

Keeping busy helped me to "forget" about the pain for a little while. I tried to stay positive, but things were truly a struggle in every way. I do not look forward to travel. My mood is mostly bland and I am often told that I am negative, even today. But I had ruled out so much and I had to continue looking for the answers. The more I looked for help, the more disheartening my outcome appeared to me.

The Depths of Despair

The more I do, the more I hurt.
The more I do, the more I hurt.
The more I do, the more I hurt.

I live my life in slow motion.
I watch every step I take.
I live my life in slow motion.
I watch every step I take.

I have deep thoughts of despair.
Will I ever be free of pain?

My sadness is overwhelming.
Will this be forever?
The hopelessness is immense.
Will permanence of this distress lead to death?

Certainly, heaven is an existence better than this.
No one has any answers.
I am in a "love trap" with my family.
My daughters adore me, my grandchildren too.
"Nana, you are my best friend" said my sweet S. age 6
I will not quit searching. This trap has kept me alive.

Guilt will not win; I am not crazy.
I have so many reasons to go on.
I will look shame in the eye.
Pain will no longer be my fear.

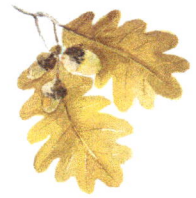

AFTER SO MANY YEARS, PERSISTENCE DIDN'T PAY OFF, IT DEPLETED ME

I was driving to get an MRI of my brain because my headaches were increasing. On the way to the imaging center, I noticed a place called "The Pain Relief Center." I had not ever put much faith in chiropractic solutions and all the doctors listed were DCs. When I got home, I looked up the clinic and sent an email to every chiropractor in the practice. I believe there were five.

#12: Dr. W, DC

The following week I got a call from Dr. W. She was very nice and caring and had a specialty in neurologic ailments. We talked and she thought she could at least help me with my headaches and possibly my sacral pain. The practice also had massage therapists and my insurance did pay for part of each visit.

I was prescribed four appointments a week. I was able to have side lying or back lying massages twice a week. I have not been able to lay prone (on abdomen) until just last year (2023). Dr. W. basically prescribed heat therapy, a TENS unit, and she attempted to adjust my neck and my sacrum, which was painful and unsuccessful on both areas every time. The massages were therapeutic, however, and I stuck with them for about six months.

At this point, Dr. W. thought that my issue must have been in one of my spinal discs. I thought, *here we go again*. The pain in my sacrum, along with instability, continued to worsen as did my feelings of exhaustion, depression, nausea, and the feeling of being poisoned was becoming extremely unsettling for me. My headaches did improve a little bit, so at least there was that. Still today, I must get neck therapy to avoid prolonged headaches. The muscles in my neck just won't forget the years of hydrocephaly when my head was much heavier.

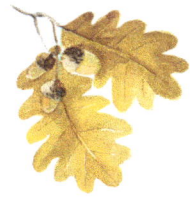

NEEDLES ANYONE?

#13: Dr. P, MD, pain management specialist

Dr. P. was a "to the point" kind of man. I brought him the MRI disc that I had from another doctor. He never ordered a new MRI for me. He was called on by the law firms to be deposed in my mesh lawsuit and he did not tell the truth. He focused on an old injury at the lumbar 5-Sacral 1 level.

I remember when Dr. P. did his initial exam on me, his emphasis was on my lower extremities and my pelvis. His son did range of motion on my lower extremities as well as "pressure-counter-pressure" type maneuvers, having me squeeze my knees, while bent, against his hands towards the middle and the lateral sides. This was an attempt to re-align my pelvis. He needed to do this at every appointment. He did not mention this in his deposition, which I believe was related to my unstable pelvis. During these maneuvers, I felt pain in my lower back and at the "joint" in my pubic bone. Dr. P, liked to treat with injections and at every appointment he injected about 10 areas along my spine. This was not terrible, but also not pleasant.

Dr. P. prescribed a medication that he said would "help me lose weight." He was more concerned about my weight than my pain. He was convinced that my problem was from the disc issue that he noticed on the MRI. I went through four outpatient surgeries for two epidural injections and one for "Pro lo therapy," which is basically injecting glucose into the damaged disc so it builds scar tissue and may perhaps strengthen that area of the spine. I will say that he was proficient, and thankfully, he gave me adequate anesthesia.

At this point, Dr. P. decided I should see a neurosurgeon who then asked Dr. P. to inject my sacroiliac joints with lidocaine to see if my pain improved. It felt a little better until the lidocaine wore off. For some reason, Dr. GW, the neurosurgeon, saw this result as a reason to fuse my Sacroiliac joints. Just like that!

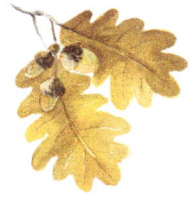

JUMP RIGHT IN! NOT

#14: Dr. G, MD, Neurosurgeon

This recommendation was a disaster right from the first time I met Dr. G. He seemed very scattered and took a quick look at my records. I was not taken to an exam room. He did not sit down with me or explain why he had decided that he should fuse my SI joints. I never felt that I was his center of attention, even for 15 seconds. I was not thrilled about having any part of my body fused.

Many neurosurgeons jump right into surgery because that is what they do, and it pays. Because the SI joints are part of my pelvis, attaching my sacrum to my ilium, which is part of my hip, made no sense to me. My pelvis was fragile, yes, but I need my SI joints to function even to the very minor amount they move. I left his office and never went back. Not surprisingly, they never got in touch with me either. There are a lot of doctors in Florida. But there are good doctors and bad doctors. Choose wisely my friends.

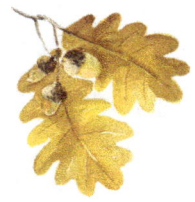

A PAINFUL STRETCH!

#15: SH, PT, I saw her for a long time

There came a time when I was unable to do the Pilates classes any-more. M, my instructor, suggested that I see her friend, S, a Physical Therapist.

S was a "Pilates-based physical therapist," and she and C, a massage therapist who worked out of the same office, really tried hard to fig-ure out why I was not getting better. Having stuck with the Pilates class for so long, unwilling to give up, I took the advice of my Pilates instructor and went to S. Her physical therapy office was based on the principles of Pilates. She had a reformer, which is the main piece of equipment in Pilates. She also worked with me on exercises and stretches that were based on the Pilates principles. She had other various pieces of equipment in her office, one being a machine you get strapped into and traction is applied to wherever necessary.

Since the problem for me was in my pelvis, it seemed appropriate for her to apply traction to the lower half of my body. This was in hopes of expanding any spinal disc area that may be flattened and causing pressure on the spinal nerves. This traction caused my low back to go into an immediate, major spasm. If you picture my sacroiliac joints already arthritic from constant rubbing on each other because of the pull of the mesh and then add a somewhat heavy weight downward, you might be able to get a sense of the response of my body. The spasm was immediate, the pain was intense, and even once the weight was taken off, I had to lay there for quite a while. Heat was applied on the front of my pelvis. After an hour or so, with many tears, I fought through the pain and forced myself to sit up and then stand with a pole and get to the heated seats of my car. I had never used my cruise control so much at a low speed as I did to and from these appointments.

At the next appointment, S decided to attack the "problem" from the back. I had not laid on my tummy (prone position) for years. In my continued desperation, I agreed that with a pillow under my hips I would try. While in this position for an hour she applied both electro-stimulation therapy and ultrasound therapy, intermittently. During the actual "hands on" part of the treatments, it felt pretty good. She then applied an ice pack to constrict the blood vessels decreasing the flow of blood to the area to decrease any swelling that had occurred, followed by heat therapy which would then dilate the blood vessels allowing fresh oxygenated blood to enter the area. S announced that the session was over and that I should slowly sit up. My first attempt of flexing my hips to get to my knees, brought on the worst spasm that I had ever experienced. I could not move. S got more pillows to help support my contracted pelvis. Eventually, I had to fight through the pain, get to my knees and slide off the edge of the table onto my feet, eliminating the step of sitting before standing. S got me a cane and I managed to slowly make it to my car.

What in the heck was going on? These people were trying their best to help me and so many had failed. This made "foul play" a clearer possibility to me. Something was impairing my body's ability to "accept" help. My body and my way of life were fading away. I decided that despite S's great intentions, and no fault of hers, I would move on from this therapy.

#16: Dr. PZ, MD, Rheumatologist, 2013-14

I waited about eight months for an appointment with Dr. PZ, the only positive rated rheumatologist in the area. She is probably in her 70s with a lot of positive reviews and years of experience. I believe I inflicted a bit of a puzzle into her diagnostic expertise.

I realized right away that Dr. PZ is extremely well-schooled in her specialty, but once I gave her my history and she had finished the exam, I could sense her perplexity mixed with true concern. I saw her once a week for the first month. She would examine me, hands on, every time. A rather rare occurrence these days especially with some primary care physicians, who will often listen to your story while deciding which specialist might fit your needs.

At each visit, Dr. PZ would check my extremities, mostly assessing any changes in the pain and swelling that I was experiencing in my hands, feet and elbows. She always found my hands swollen, as did I each morning since after the mesh was implanted. Many joints were always swollen and tender and she injected them with cortisone at a couple of visits. My feet hurt in general with Plantar Fasciitis being extremely troubling over the last of those years and still today. Regarding Plantar Fasciitis, I learned a lot, that I describe later in the section titled, "origins and insertions."

Dr. PZ prescribed five medications, one at a time. These were mostly new experimental drugs. At this point, I knew something crazy was going on in my body, but I still had not connected it to the mesh. After trying four medications, and having them do nothing to help me, Dr. PZ asked if I would try Methotrexate, which is a chemotherapy drug. Reluctantly, I took it for 12 weeks with no changes. Dr. PZ became more and more perplexed. As I was working with her, I was also concluding that I had tried all possible treatment modalities.

The next trial drug Dr. PZ prescribed was Lyrica. This is a "nerve pain relief" medicine, which seemed to help early on. This was a new and expensive drug even with insurance. I had been having numb-ness and tingling of my hands and feet for a while and the Lyrica seemed to help. Lyrica was not supposed to be habit-forming, but I believe it was the hardest medication I have ever weaned myself from. It had other side effects as do all medications. At times, I didn't know if what I was feeling was a result of my "illness" or the drugs I was taking.

Talking to my sister, she told me a friend of hers who had good relief from post radiation nerve pain, by taking vitamin B6 (two tabs a day) continuously, needing a few weeks to feel the effects. The dose was higher, but it did work. Adding these inflammatory issues as well as many "trial" medications to my list of ailments and treat-ments brought me to an even lower place in my life. I was now hang-ing heavily from that branch on the live oak, but it was getting much harder to hold on. Taking so many pills does increase heartburn for me, GERD, (gastroesophageal reflux disease) and then I need the drug Nexium, which reduces acid. I just couldn't win this war.

Dr. PZ wanted to do a trial of oral prednisone, for a four-day course. I was hesitant because this is a steroid which will suppress the im-mune system. However! It was only for four days. I agreed and, in the end, this was the only medication that gave me any relief at all over the course of these past five years of suffrage.

It was only two days, but two days of hope! Something that I had not felt in a very long time. Two whole days of feeling like I could do just a little more around the house and not pay for it with a debili-tating spike in pain and spasms by day's end. Blood tests to measure inflammation in the body were elevated for me. This told Dr. P. that I had, *and still have*, significant inflammation in my body.

Unfortunately, it is dangerous to stay on steroids long term. Dr. PZ allowed me two "bursts" (four days in a row) of prednisone, over the next few months so I might be more comfortable attending two wedding events. That was great until I developed sores inside my nose that would not heal. Of course, as I always do, I called my daughters, one who is a nurse practitioner and the other a certified registered nurse anesthetist. From their advice, I knew I had to stop the prednisone. I have never gone back on any systemic steroids. *I believe my immune system to be less than strong.*

I spent a lot of time with Dr. PZ because she really felt that I had an autoimmune disease other than Hashimoto's Thyroiditis. My diagnosis included the words "non-sero," meaning it did not show up in my blood studies. Having all these lab studies done and trying so many different medications, with no positive outcomes or explanations brought me to the point, where I pulled myself up onto the branch of the live oak tree and decided that if things did not improve during the summer in Maine, where we were soon heading, I would call Dr. M, who had implanted the mesh in 2009 and request for him to remove it.

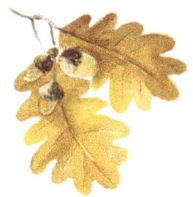

THE PRESSURE IS BUILDING!
I MUST ACT

The television was on, as it often was. I watched a lot of television series and I read many books, in the five years that I can only describe as torture. I remained in my bed most of the time leading up to that summer. My husband remembers. There was nothing more he or I could do here in Saint Augustine to help me. There was no one else to see. I was out on the tip of that branch. And on this day, I decided to take action that would either prove myself right or wrong.

"Courage isn't having the strength to go on, it is going on when you don't have the strength."
—NAPOLEON BONAPARTE

I had seen the commercials. They kept stressing that if anyone had mesh implanted as part of a gynecologic surgery, that they should contact the lawyer on the screen. At that moment, in all my desperation and physical anguish watching gray squirrels race around my tree, I decided I was going to call around to several lawyers who were advertising online as taking on clients who have mesh issues and then, once in Maine, if I did not get any relief, I would call my surgeon, Dr. M.

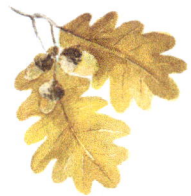

MAINE, "THE WAY LIFE SHOULD BE"

On Father's Day of 2014, my surgeon, Dr. M. returned my call of desperation. I finally was getting through to him that I was in serious trouble. I was in bed on a beautiful day and was quite impressed that he called on this holiday. I did my best to give him the shortest version possible of the past five years, and the myriad of approaches I had taken to find out why I was becoming increasingly ill and incapacitated.

Dr. M. told me that if I went for an appointment with his colleague, Dr. F, whom he went to the University of New England with, and if If I got a bone scan to rule out an infection in my sacrum, he would look at the possibility of doing the removal surgery. The bone scan was replaced by a different scan in which they take blood on one day, spin it down to separate the white blood cells out, and then upon my return the next day, they inject only the white blood cells back into my body, it would then show on an x-ray if there was anything going on in my sacrum. The result was that it showed "activity bilaterally." But no osteomyelitis. I was able to get an appointment with Dr. F. within two weeks.

#16: Dr. F, Urogynecology
July 2, 2014-Oct 23,2014

My husband and I went together to meet Dr. F on the first visit. He assured us that the mesh was not causing my pelvic instability or my ongoing urinary discomfort and urethritis (painful urination due to inflammation of the urethral opening). He decided that I had "interstitial cystitis," this was the same diagnosis that K, the NP from my PCP in Florida, had bestowed upon me as she hurried me out the door of the new urogynecology office where she now worked.

(I had made an appointment last minute to see if she could do an exam and confirm if there was mesh erosion in my vaginal canal. She told me I did not have mesh erosion, and handed me a pamphlet on IC on the way out of the office).

After 12 office visits with Dr. F, laying in the most uncomfortable position, flat on my low back feet in stirrups, I was waiting for bladder installations via urinary catheter, which I was to hold in my bladder for as long as possible after leaving the office. Along with this, to treat my non-gyn problem, he prescribed two rounds of antibiotics for a urinary tract infection. The only sense this makes to me is the reason he quit that job shortly after my last visit and moved to The Villages in Florida, where he was the doctor in charge, to be behind a desk where he should have been.

Why are most Gynecologists men anyway? I can only guess because women were not allowed to practice medicine until the mid 1800s and I am sure those first women physicians were not well-received. It took many years before women were given the credit they deserve for being smart and at the same level as any male doctor.

On my last visit with Dr. F, he decided my problem was not at all to do with gynecology. I was still taking urinary pain pills almost daily and my life was like that of a limp rag doll. Dr. F told me on my last visit that he did not think I had interstitial cystitis, for which I had 12 extremely uncomfortable bladder installations. Dr. F finally passed the buck by suggesting I return to my rheumatologist once back in Florida. I had no respect for this man.

Before "going under the knife" as some say, I decided to get the opinion of Dr B, the neurosurgeon who operated on my brain, to rule out any spinal issues that could be causing my pain. I had zero trust in the neurosurgeon I saw in Florida.

We stayed in Maine and I consulted with Dr. B, my brain surgeon. I had to go around his 'brick wall" of physician's assistants, who absolutely would not allow me even a phone appointment with Dr. B because my MRI, which I mailed to them, was not in their opinion, a surgical issue. Thank God that the man who did my brain surgery was compassionate to me and arranged me to see Dr. NB. I am so thankful for Dr. B, my neurosurgeon, and Dr. NB for finally believing what I was suffering from.

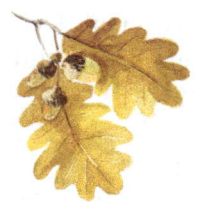

THANK YOU, GOD! SOMEONE BELIEVES ME!

#17: Dr. NB, MD, 2014, neuro rehab in the same practice with Dr. B, neurosurgeon.

Dr. NB is a very professional, kind and real doctor. She looked at my MRI, showed me where my past injury had healed, sat down with me and looked at a social media site for mesh survivors. Dr. NB referred me to the best pelvic floor physical therapist in the area. Someone was finally seeing where my problem was.

#18: Dr. A, DPT

Dr. A. worked with me on both the core work, which at least stretched my long muscles, and on the vaginal, urethral pain issues, I tried many techniques to calm the vulvodynia down. But in the end, Dr. A. told me I needed to get the mesh removed. With all this information, Dr. M. agreed to see me and plan for at least an exploratory surgery.

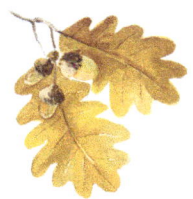

HANGING ON TO THE TRUNK OF THE LIVE OAK TREE, FINALLY!

When we got back to Florida in November of 2014, I scheduled surgery with Dr. M. I would arrive in Atlanta on Dec 8th for my pre-op evaluation and then, if needed, proceed to surgery on Dec 9, 2014.

I had the mesh removal surgery. During my pre-op exam, Dr. M knew and voiced that the mesh was being stretched and it was tight. The following morning after the removal, Dr. M checked on me and told me that it was "a big surgery." I told him I already felt some relief

He told me that a lot of women feel that at first, but I should be prepared for a lengthy recovery. He also told me that he had only removed around 50 of the Y slings and about 500 of the mini slings. The mesh could not only have been on its way through my vaginal wall, but common sense told me that this polypropylene could be breaking down, releasing chemicals that were making me feel constantly queasy, as well as causing the ever-worsening pelvic instability that had stolen my ambitions, my activities, my ability to devote time to my loved ones and so much more.

In 2019, the FDA pulled some of the mesh devices off the market, but not all.

My removal surgery was a success in that most of the mesh was removed. A piece near a large blood vessel could not be removed. The scar tissue is here to stay. My life will never be the same, but I am blessed to be alive and to hopefully help others through this book.

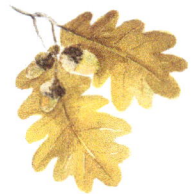

LEGAL DISAPPOINTMENTS

I would never have thought in my life that I would consider myself disabled. Until my sister pointed out to me that I had worked for 30 years, and now because of the mesh invading and taking my body over, I can no longer work.

I was denied disability three times, after the first time I got a lawyer. He didn't cost me anything. He really tried to help me. He gave me the feeling that it was a slam dunk because I had so many medical records from my other lawsuit. So, per his advice, I didn't say much, I didn't tell my story. This was during COVID, and my lawyer did not want to do an online hearing. I would have. Just to get it done. So, we waited.

Finally, we got another in-person meeting scheduled and my lawyer got covid. The third time I was so prepared to talk about my nursing career and my problems with pelvic mesh. He denied me again. I wrote a letter to the judge (see next page), which I doubt he will ever see, letting him know about how debilitating mesh can be and so to please keep an open mind when considering people who go from wanting to work hard to not being able to do anything. Except "walk on the beach" and so I chose to take my social security benefit early and get on with my life. I really could not write this book until all legal matters were settled. I have wanted to write this book since 2013. I want to help other women who are suffering and may not realize why.

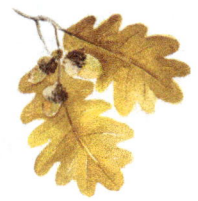

SHOULD NON-MEDICAL JUDGES & LAWYERS BE THE DECISION-MAKERS FOR PEOPLE WITH MEDICAL PROBLEMS? I THINK NOT.

Below is a slightly revised letter that I wrote to the judge who denied my request for disability.

Three times. I tried repeatedly to prove that I was a hard worker and had worked for 30 years as a nurse. I expressed how I had endured many hardships and returned to work even after becoming a widow, single mom and after having brain surgery.

> *Hello, my name is Diane May Ritter-Gardner.*
>
> *I received a notice of unfavorable decision from the Office of Hearing operations. Judge H was my judge for 2 hearings.*
>
> *I really feel the need to pass on some information, some of which pertains directly to me but an article that talks about a woman in Australia, who pretty much had the same symptoms as me for the small bladder sling mesh, she did not have the larger*

"sacrocolpopexy Y shaped mesh that I had implanted in 2009 and most of it removed in 2014.

Once I started looking around online, I noticed that there are far more women who are speaking out because they have suffered, like me, for years. I believe there are most likely many others who are suffering in silence not knowing what is causing them pain and the many other side effects of poly propylene mesh. This "PVC" plastic mesh, used in hysterectomies to "take the place" of the uterus in holding up the woman's organs. There are some men as well who have had reactions to the mesh after a hernia repair.

Back in 2014 once I finally had gone to 28 doctors, (MD'S, DOs, DCs, acupuncturist) and also 7 therapists because of relationship issues and self-worth issues, seven physical therapists and about 15 different massage therapists trying desperately to find an answer to my disabling pain and pelvic instability.

I do believe that I could find evidence in my medical records that would possibly be "exceptions" to the reasons Judge H thought valid to make an unfavorable decision. But what I really want to do here is make it known that women are suffering from this mesh which is still used. They present with pelvic pain and instability, hip pain, back pain, multiple urinary tract infections, stress, urinary incontinence, painful sexual relations and like me they or their doctors can't find any reasons or helpful treatments.

Patients who are adult women most likely have had babies and some have jobs they cannot just quit. Even today if someone asks me "how are you" I must stop and think about whether I want to burden that person with the truth. I have not felt "good" since 2009 in regard to being able to function as a woman my age should. I had to stop working in 2010. (I may have helped them out with an immunization clinic in 2011)? I was working Per diem as an RN in their student health center. I have not been able to work since then.

For five years, I suffered as my pain and fragility of my pelvis increased as well as having a feeling of being poisoned and I felt that some doctors did not believe me, they thought I was a drug seeker, or a hypochondriac.

Those 5 years were the worst of my life, and I was widowed at age 33 having 3 daughters under 10. I also had brain surgery after years of debilitating headaches, which I had to work through.

In regard to the mesh, I was misdiagnosed several times which got me lots of painful spinal injections and "bladder instillations" for "Interstitial Cystitis" which I didn't have. And after 5 years and even today some of my family definitely have "compassion fatigue." It is a life of despair and limitations for me even now.

For five years, I pretty much stayed in bed unless I had an appointment. I lived my life in slow motion, and I still do today, thankfully to a lesser degree, since there is still some mesh in my sacrum and every now and then if I step the wrong way, on an uneven surface, my sacrum will spasm. I still have a feeling of being poisoned with nausea and fatigue.

I hope this letter will offer the courts the knowledge that some people truly are in pain but trying desperately to live a life and move forward.

Thank you for your time,

Respectfully, Diane Ritter-Gardner RN, BSN

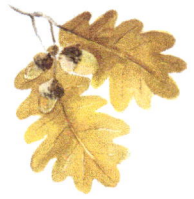

ORIGINS & INSERTIONS

A rather infuriating fact came to mind in the height of my chronic foot pain, *because I have taught Anatomy and Physiology*, and I know that when treating plantar fasciitis, one must massage *aggressively* from the **origin** of the Achilles tendon to its **insertion** point, which lies deep in the middle of the calf muscles. One of the chiropractors that I specifically asked to treat this painful condition seemed to not know the cause, or the connection to the Achilles tendon. A, my massage therapist, later that same day, in her own office, gave me much relief with this approach to treating plantar fasciitis. Wearing Birkenstocks has also curbed my foot pain.

Polypropylene mesh continues to change the direction and the goals for my life. This book is part of what I hope will be a new beginning to help other women. I have looked at websites and social media pages specific to mesh survivors. The site I looked at with Dr. N. no longer exists. Many have not had any activity since 2020. It was 2019 when the FDA finally looked at and banned certain mesh kits. I now know that some women with mesh in their bodies are just too ill to join any online support groups. I spent most of 2012-2014 bedridden except for appointments, which did me no good.

Today, I am part of one of many social media support groups for women who are suffering in so many ways because of mesh. My heart goes out to them. The nursing education that I got in my three-year diploma school was so valuable even if I only used it to raise my family and take care of myself.

I learned things in Microbiology and Anatomy and Physiology that made such sense that it baffles me why scientists would mix two substances, human tissue and plastic, and expect it to be okay. It is like oil and water. They will not mix, the oil pulls away, much like the mesh was doing in my body. As you can see in my pathology report.

All the mesh pieces that were removed had tissue attached to them. Some was skeletal muscle tissue. Some had sutures (most likely polypropylene (plastic non absorbable) sutures still attached. There was also, "adipose tissue with a foreign body giant cell reaction." Thankfully, not malignant. I wonder if these surgeons would implant mesh in their loved ones. If they did any "homework" at all, they most definitely would not.

Final Pathologic Diagnosis
A.   'SACRAL COLPOPEXY MESH.' EXCISION:
          - SYNTHETIC MESH-LIKE MATERIAL WITH ATTACHED FIBROCONNECTIVE
   ADIPOSE TISSUE AND A FOREIGN
               BODY-TYPE GIANT CELL REACTION.
          - NO MALIGNANCY IS IDENTIFIED.

B.   'SLING MESH,' EXCISION.
          - SYNTHETIC MESH-LIKE MATERIAL WITH ATTACHED FIBROCONNECTIVE
   SKELETAL MUSCLE.
          - NO MALIGNANCY IS IDENTIFIED.

Electronically Signed Out

Clinical History
Mesh complications, dyspareunia, vaginal pain, sling pain,
urinary frequency, positive obstructive symptoms, mesh
preservation

Specimen(s) Received
A: Sacral colpexy meshS14-27654
B: Sling meshS14-27654

Gross Description
The specimen is received in two parts.

Specimen A is received in formalin labeled 'Ritter-Gardner, Diane
May' and 'sacral colpopexy mesh.' It consists of three irregular
portions of clear mesh-like material which have a small amount of
adherent cauterized tan-pink soft tissue. These portions of mesh
along with soft tissue range from 3.2 x 1.0 x 0.5 cm to 5.0 x 3 5
x 0.5 cm. Some of these portions of tissue have associated green
suture material. A portion of the soft tissue is placed in block
A1 for routine processing.

Specimen B is received in formalin labeled 'Ritter-Gardner, Diane
May' and 'sling mesh.' It consists of two elongate strips of
clear mesh-like material which average 5.5 x 0.5 x 0.1 cm. Each
portion of mesh-like material has a small amount of adherent

==cauterized pink soft tissue==. A portion of the soft tissue is submitted in block B1 for routine processing.

This case is reviewed with ▓▓▓▓▓▓▓ and is held in the Pathology Lab.

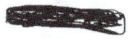

Microscopic Description
Microscopic examination supports the above diagnoses. There is no evidence of malignancy.

The interpretation of this case was performed at ▓▓▓▓▓▓▓ Hospital - ▓▓▓▓▓▓▓

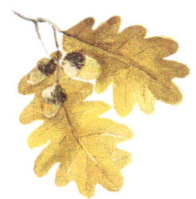

LET'S PROTECT OURSELVES & OUR REPRODUCTIVE ORGANS

Accidents happen. Or some of us just make the wrong choices.

When I think of reasons why the female body is so prone to prolapsed organs, it isn't hard to figure it out. I cannot even imagine having five children by vaginal birth (I had three) never mind having more! My hope is that any mom giving birth to any number of babies should take excellent care of herself before and after these births.

Childbirth is not only one of the most painful "activities" women perform, but it also stresses the entire body and weakens the pelvic floor muscles, creating an environment within the body that could easily exacerbate the prolapsing of organs. I still can't understand why men physicians stepped in somewhere in history and decided childbirth should take place against gravity with the laboring mom lying on her back. No wonder babies had to be hauled out with forceps while she was anesthetized with gas. That is not good for the uterine ligaments, the pelvic floor, the mother, or the baby. If you look back in history, laboring women's instincts are to be on all fours, or holding onto a bed post or a tree and stretching backwards, eventually leading to a squat, side lying or whatever position works best for her.

I was present for two of my grandbaby's births. My daughters used all the natural tools in their toolbox to allow gravity to help nature take its course. Healthy babies today are born in a totally different way than my daughters were born, and my daughters were born in a totally different way than I was born.

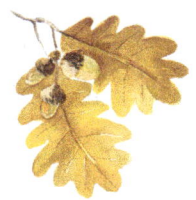

WHAT CAUSES AUTOIMMUNE DISEASES? SOME ARE GENETIC, SOME ARE NOT

The Beauty of a BM. Potty talk is popular with the young and the old.

I believe my organs prolapsed mostly from years of straining with chronic constipation caused by opioids prescribed for the relentless headaches that led me to brain surgery. I only wish someone had enlightened me to the world of magnesium oxide, much earlier than they did. I used to take other magnesium supplements and MiraLAX every day, but the results were often crampy and uncomfortable.

If you have never heard of Leaky Gut syndrome, I believe it might help you understand, in part, how autoimmune diseases work. It did for me. If a bunch of "excrement" is "stuck" in your gut, as in chronic constipation, it can decay and allow toxins to possibly pass into your blood stream through the intestinal walls. Your body sees these toxins as foreign. Our immune system attacks the toxins but at the same time it may attack healthy tissues, especially over time, for example your thyroid gland. It might be worth looking it up. I found it informational because I had chronic constipation. Pelvic organ prolapses alter the natural placement of our anatomy. This too can cause constipation.

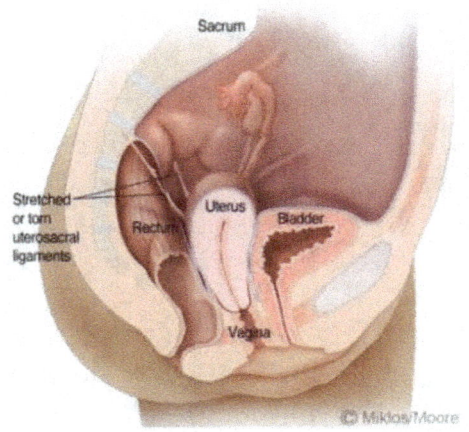

Prolapse uterus

Some women will self-treat and manipulate the pathway that is blocked, by redirecting the formed stool by pulling things back in place. Self-manipulation with a gloved thumb and forefinger attempts to do what a "pessary" would do. A pessary is a *temporary* fix and is shaped like a rubber donut. When pushed up into the top of the vagina, around the cervix, from the outside of our body, it helps hold falling organs in place. If people understood the human body, by teaching children from the very first grade, I believe many injuries and illnesses could be prevented, not to mention STDs and unplanned pregnancies.

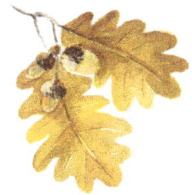

STRONG IN WILL,
STUBBORN IN MIND

We women are strong and sometimes stubborn. Self-motivation and ambitious goals can get women into serious trouble if not done wisely and carefully. My friend L is in her element when she is moving rocks around to change up her landscape and garden. I am pleased when she uses a fulcrum like a crowbar, but her excitement for the project and determination to get it done "yesterday" could be causing her harm.

Men tend to use heavy accessories like 30-pound "come-a-longs" to move heavier things (less chance of them getting a hernia), and then some don't, like my father-in-law who insisted, years ago, that my mother-in-law get on one side of a roof truss and help move it. I wish she had been strong in mind at that occurrence. I wish she would have said, "NO, sorry." She landed in the operating room having her prolapsed organs repaired. Men are built differently with larger muscles throughout their bodies. We should try to let them use those muscles to help us not damage our bodies, or lower the expectations we have for ourselves physically.

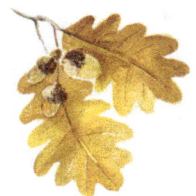

BLACK-LEGGED DEER TICKS

Yuck! Lyme disease, autoimmune disease? Good question.

Lyme disease has become a major health concern for our population. It is caused by a bacterium which is carried by the black-legged deer tick. The nymphs of these arthropods, which are as tiny as a pinhead, are often not even noticed, they do the actual biting. The bullseye rash that may develop later is much more visible.

Although it is not considered an autoimmune disease, Lyme disease symptoms are often like other autoimmune diseases. It is also not easy to diagnose as there was not much faith put in the three different and rather expensive blood tests that I have gone through twice. The first test was negative. The NP I was seeing at the time, in 2012, did not like that answer so she wanted me to have a second test for Lyme. Also, negative. Ten years later, now with a DO as my NP, I did it all again. Maybe because I had been back in Maine where there are a lot of deer? So after the third blood test, again, $500 (I guess not much has changed with the testing protocol since the cost is the same?), but the results were the same. Negative on all three tests.

The PCP that I was seeing, here in Maine in 2022, did not seem to believe the test results. This was all very confusing because she still wanted me to seek treatment with a naturopath (not sure of his credentials), who required a $250 down payment just to make an appointment. I did not believe it made sense to pay a practitioner before I even met him. I also felt that between having had brain surgery and polypropylene mesh in my body in varying amounts since 2009, that my symptoms which include headaches, sacral, and other joint pain, fatigue and a few more, were most likely a result of my past medical history.

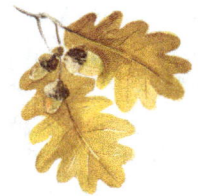

PROBABLY IN OUR FAMILY
FOR YEARS, CELIAC

C eliac disease is another autoimmune disease that affects our gastrointestinal system. For me, it showed negative on one biopsy of my small intestine during a scoped procedure, but positive on a blood test (identified by one of the protein markers).

My sister and two of her daughters have Celiac and have been miserable for quite some time. The only way to control it is to avoid wheat. You would not believe how many foods and sauces have wheat. I also don't digest dairy products well. Many of these autoimmune diseases do not show up until adulthood, which makes sense because our bodies, in some cases, take years to build up the "army" of self-attacking, illness-provoking cells. There are many more autoimmune diseases in which our body's own immune systems attack healthy tissues in various organs and body systems. Celiac can cause constipation or diarrhea. If you have concerns, get tested.

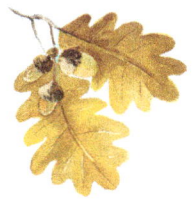

FIBROMYALGIA SYNDROME,
AUTOIMMUNE DISEASE

During a massage, the padded, heated surface helps with comfort, but I usually needed to follow it with ice. The heat feels so good and increases the diameter of the vessels (dilatates), which brings in more oxygen and healing nutrients.

It also brings in fluid, which increases swelling and inflammation. Ice comes to the rescue for the first 48 hours when dealing with an acute injury. Cold constricts the tiny vessels, which pushes fluid out of the cells allowing the vessels to get ready for their next batch of oxygenated blood. White blood cells carry away any damaged or dead cells, when they do the switch, with the oxygenated blood.

In Fibromyalgia, everywhere you push on a person's body hurts. This includes mine. I was diagnosed by Dr. PZ, qualifying the diagnosis with the criteria necessary for "fibromyalgia syndrome," during one of our final visits in 2014. It is now defined in Wikipedia, as "a medical condition defined by the presence of chronic widespread pain, fatigue, weight gain, cognitive symptoms, lower abdominal pain or cramps." "Fibro" as my Rheumatologist called it, is also associated with depression. *Honestly, what isn't?*

The cause of fibromyalgia is unknown. It originated in the 1940s. It is believed to involve a combination of genetic and environmental factors, such as psychological stress, trauma, and certain infections. That sure sounds like me and, most likely, a lot of readers. The symptoms include insomnia and a general hypersensitivity to light, sounds, touch, smells and tastes. From memories of my nursing experience, fibromyalgia has not been recognized adequately by some practitioners, especially in years past. Thankfully, now it is known and there are treatments available. Self-care being the one I chose although that is not always easy.

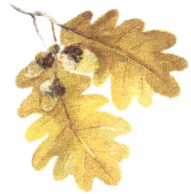

WHY DID I WRITE THIS BOOK?

My surgeon told me that "less than 1% of women, who have mesh placed during surgery, in the world, will have mesh complications." Lucky Me! According to Premierhealth. com, in the United States alone, approximately 600,000 hysterectomies are performed every year. Assuming mesh was used, since it *was* the gold standard for so many years for these surgeries, that would mean that each year, 6,000 women could, and I believe most likely would, develop some type of mesh complications. It is also written in this article that hysterectomies are one of the most common surgeries performed in the U.S., second only to cesarean sections.

In an article by myclevelandclinic.org, it states that in 2010 one in three women, who had pelvic organ prolapse repairs, had surgical mesh implanted. This would be the larger Y sling that invaded my entire pelvic cavity. I will share the list of pre-operative and post-operative complications that I developed over the five years of misery that I endured. Also 80% of women who had surgery for SUI in 2010 had the mini sling implanted.

Revision/ Removal

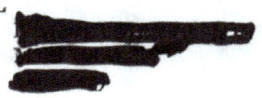

OPERATIVE NOTE
NORTHSIDE HOSPITAL

DATE: ~~████~~ 2014

PATIENT: ~~██████~~ Diane ~~████████~~

PREOPERATIVE DIAGNOSES:
1. Vaginal pain.
2. Urinary obstructive symptoms.
3. Dyspareunia.
4. Pelvic pain.
5. Back pain.
6. Mesh complication.
7. Mesh contraction. .
8. Severe pain on palpation of both sling mesh and sacrocolpopexy mesh.
9. Contraction and bunching of her apical mesh.
10. Retroperitoneal fibrosis.
11. Pelvic adhesions.

POSTOPERATIVE DIAGNOSES:
1. Vaginal pain.
2. Urinary obstructive symptoms.
3. Dyspareunia.
4. Pelvic pain.
5. Back pain.
6. Mesh complication.
7. Mesh contraction.
8. Severe pain on palpation of both sling mesh and sacrocolpopexy mesh.
9. Contraction and bunching of her apical mesh.
10. Retroperitoneal fibrosis.
11. Pelvic adhesions.

OPERATION:
1. Sling revision/removal (entire mini sling including self-fixating tips).
2. Right ureteral stent placement.
3. Laparoscopic adhesiolysis.
4. Laparoscopic right ureterolysis.
5. Laparoscopic sacrocolpopexy mesh removal.
6. Laparoscopic uterosacral vault suspension.
7. Cystoscopy.
8. Urethrolysis.

SURGEON: ~~████████~~

The media presents many different facts and numbers on how many women have problems. Honestly, I wonder how a woman can have *plastic* mesh forced into the walls of her vagina and not have problems. I also wonder how many women don't realize that they even have mesh in their vaginal walls or pelvic cavity. After all, I am a nurse of 43 years and I did not know That I had the mini sling mesh inside my vaginal walls until six years after it was implanted. It caused an immense amount of struggle in my life as well as pain, that I pretty much ignored and endured "chalking it up" to trauma caused by the hysterectomy. The larger Y mesh was pulling on my sacrum and I could in no way ignore the instability and spasms that prevented my activities of daily living.

I was trying to find a way to make life comfortable and fulfilling again for myself and my husband. I thank God for him every day because he stood by me when many men, according to social media blogs and such, just walked away. How horribly cruel and devastating for these women who did not know, like me, *hanging onto that tiny live oak branch*, wondering which way they should go next. Some, I am guessing, did not continue the pursuit. They gave up and tolerated their worsening condition and either died or now have ostomy bags outside of their bodies into which the excrement of bowels and bladder go. The outcomes are horrendous.

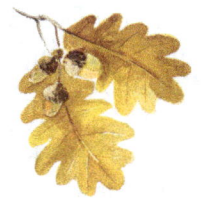

PREVENTION IS KEY, KNOWLEDGE IS EVERYTHING

I want to stress so strongly that there are ways out. The first is to never get in that position. Prevention, in my opinion, is key. Find out what your surgeon is planning on doing. Avoid polypropylene mesh or any other synthetic material to be put in your body.

My organs are now being held up by my own uterine ligaments. Even after five years of just "hanging around," they were still healthy and strong enough to do the job. Oh, how I wish my doctor had just done that in the beginning. I would not have this constant pain and burning in the left side of my sacrum and across my low back area into my hips. The old way is sometimes the better way.

Women also need to know that they can have surgical intervention, even if the surgeon starts with one or two small incisions and does an "exploratory lap," in which they use a scope to go inside and see what is happening with the mesh and your organs. They can then decide from there how to proceed. There are surgeons out there who do care and do want to help, if this is all new to you, the prolapse, the incontinence. Why not try some non-surgical options, which were never offered to me, at least until you have more information and feel strong enough to move ahead to a more final solution.

I should have taken responsibility and asked for a pessary. But most women don't know what a pessary is. Surgeons like to operate. So if you are referred to a surgeon, most likely they will suggest surgery. We need to be brave and seek help. We need to look after other women, our mothers, sisters, grandmothers, friends and daughters. And men as well since mesh has been used to repair inguinal hernias since the 1800s. I would venture to guess that the materials used back then were not plastic, but these men still had reactions to cotton or wool or whatever was tried. I wonder if infection was more the culprit at that time.

Mesh has been used widely for a long time and has not been the focus of enough attention. Finally, it is being brought into the light. Who was the "*genius*" that decided to take a non-biodegradable plastic and turn it into a medical product used in the human body? These "scientists," as they refer to themselves, came up with a way to make things easier on surgeons, and perhaps in many of the cases, the mesh was implanted, and the patients did fine. Or did they? Women are particularly tough. We endure, suffer, get through, and tolerate pain and inconveniences in our lives. Since long ago, women have worked their *asses* off, doing whatever needed to be done to keep the household running.

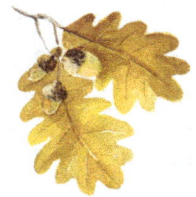

SUPPORT IS AVAILABLE

One social media site that I am a member of has over 10,000 members. There are currently many sites which you must be allowed to join. In one country there was a study that concluded that of the total number of mesh products implanted, a very high percentage of those products had been removed.

The cries for help break my heart. Some may have waited too long; some are not aware that they have mesh inside of their body. Some will perforate a bowel because of mesh erosion and if untreated could die. Some have zero control of their bladder and must wear special undergarments all the time. I have wanted to be as much help as possible because, although the CDC has banned some mesh products, they have not banned them all. Will hospitals just throw away "perfectly good mesh?" Are they or were they buying mesh products on eBay? As I saw? I believe it possible that the non-medical person in charge would see this as throwing money out the window.

Also, unfortunately, our healthcare system has become dominated by the rules of insurance companies. Insurance people who know nothing about human anatomy or health are making life changing decisions for people they do not know. It seems to me that it has an awful lot to do with money. They have no right to decide what is put in our bodies. We must read and understand everything that is happening to us in any surgery. We need to take back control of our bodies and our heath!

Paraphrased excerpts from social media sites.

So many women tell the same story. Doctors will not listen. The pharmaceutical companies are making billions of dollars. While we are left to suffer.

- *I have no bladder control. The doctors don't even want to know.*
- *I have told many different nurses and doctors that I can feel the mesh cutting into me. None of them believe me.*
- *I feel every movement of the broken off mesh. It is coming through my skin. My private parts and my buttocks like splinters. Some of them I pull out of me with tweezers. But they are so fragile they break with each touch.*
- *I send many of my patients for hernia repairs. Many of them return. With the mesh not working causing them pain, inflammation, and an area that is not healed.*
- *In the middle of all of this pain, members of social media websites take the time to wish each other a happy new year.*
- *The ability for these people to interject humor into their suffering amazes me. Mostly women are on the sites. But there are a few men.*
- *I am so happy there are other women, who understand what I mean. Thank you.*
- *If I had to do it again, I would go with mesh made from pigs. I understand they are genetically close to us.*
- *I was awake for the 4th night, struggling with nerve pain, I want to rip my leg off.*
- *I was told "you have just lost your mojo."*

- Several women talk about feeling a vibration both before and after mesh removal, they check their cell phones, near their hips, and groin area. They have found out it is caused by nerve damage from the mesh.

- I would like to join this group. I have a mini sling type mesh and am always in pain.

- From a man who had a hernia repair. I chose to have a Bassini repair, not mesh, which was good 100 years before mesh came along. Other men I know who had mesh are waiting to have it removed.

- I have fibromyalgia which developed after having a mesh repair.

- My vaginal suppositories are ending up in my bladder.

- It is so difficult to come to terms with the inability to have a normal life.

- After a party very close to home, couldn't get the key to work, embarrassed to the end of the earth.

- I am going to end up dying or on dialysis. There is no one who can help me.

- Two mesh implants without consent. One in 2005, one in 2009. I am suffering from rectal damage; vaginal infections and I wear pampers 24/7.

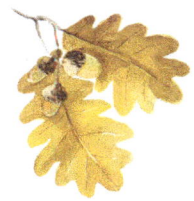

LAW FIRMS &
INSURANCE COMPANIES

In the seventh year of my lawsuit, I was given a third offer from the mesh manufacturer of $200,000. My legal counsel group, of which I had three different lawyers and seven different paralegals over seven years, encouraged me to take the offer. The head of the team explained that of several women she represented in court in mesh cases, she won *none of their cases*. I was told I could expect to get half of the $200,000.

This was, like I said, year seven. I needed to end this so I could write this book. I accepted the offer. I knew the law firm would get 40%. I assumed, and yes, I know what they say about assuming, but I was done. Well, I got the "butt end" of that deal (pun intended). The 40% did not include all the extras like phone calls, emails, texts, snail mail, storing the mesh pieces for seven years, my train tickets to my deposition plus lodging, and more.

I got a check for $28,000. I had been driving my 2002 highlander for 20 years. With the 28k, I traded my highlander for a 2017 MKC Lincoln with heated seats and a heated steering wheel. My lawyer had told me that they would hold back $50,000 in case someone claimed that I owed them money. She also mentioned that she has never had any company or doctor's office take any of the money that had been set aside in other cases. I did not owe anyone money. The very large insurance company who covered only one of my surgeries, decided that they were entitled to all the money set aside.

My Philadelphia law firm now had a different lawyer contact me because my former lawyer changed to a different firm. This "new" lawyer told me that he did not agree with this action by the insurance company. He told me that they had met with this insurance company's lawyers to go over the statistics, and that there was "nothing more they could do."

The initial check of $28,000 was for the pain and suffering I had endured, not for medical bills. I wrote a personal letter to this insurance company, trying to understand why they felt they were owed any money. (copy of letter in back of book.) I never heard back. There are times when I still want to talk to a different law firm about this because it seems to me that either the law firm is in cahoots with the insurance company, or the law firm decided that they did not receive enough payment for their services and perhaps just kept my money? I was not taxed on money received for pain and suffering. I wonder if whoever ended up with my money will claim it as taxable income.

Dear Sir or Madam: Feb 22, 2021

My name is Diane Ritter-Gardner,

I have been working with a law firm " XxxxxxXxxxxxx" for nearly 7 years trying to regain some of the income that I lost (roughly $600,000 (if I worked 24 hrs a week as an RN) because I was part of the unlucky 1% of women who reacted poorly to the surgical mesh that was implanted in my body. My first surgery was in 2009. This is when the mesh was implanted. I had 2 types. One was attached to my sacrum (the bone of the spine above the tailbone) holding up the remaining organs after the removal of my uterus. Starting a month or so after this surgery, I started having significant low back pain and pelvic instability. This pain increased as time went on and my life was lived in very slow motion to avoid sudden spasm and immobility. I still suffer that fate though to a lesser degree. The other mesh was a tiny piece that was burrowed into my vaginal wall to help combat "stress urinary incontinence". I am embarrassed to say that I did not even know this was put in for several years after the surgery) What this mesh did was cause me chronic Urinary tract infections and a life changing turn in my marriage in general. I have been a nurse for 40 years. I tried to go back to work after the surgery (the mesh that was attached to my sacrum was holding up my organs because there was a void where my uterus had been. Both types of mesh are still used today. I did not know why my back was so unstable. I could not even bend down to put an ace bandage on a patient without severe spasm and the inability to stand up. I only lasted 2 semesters at a College in health services). For 5 years I went to 30+ practitioners from massage therapists to orthopedic surgeons. (This doctor wanted to fuse my sacral iliac joints! I did not go back to him) Your company helped me pay for many of these practitioners. Many were not covered by insurance. I was desperate. Unable to work, unable to provide the monetary support that we had planned on to get us to a place where my husband could retire. He worked for "An insurance group as a Safety engineer for 34 years, retired and is now working for a construction company as their safety person.) Because my late husband of 13 years was military, I did not have longevity at any one job. In the 13 years he served, we lived in 7 places and have 3 wonderful daughters. I had no real retirement benefits.

For many years you provided medical insurance to my husband and myself. Mostly me since my husband has had minimal health concerns in his life. I, on the other hand have had a few. I got hit by a car and nearly died at age 8 from head trauma, I had headaches from unknown hydrocephaly for years which also stressed my neck and led to emergency brain surgery in 1999 and then the mesh which still haunts me today. We changed our insurance sometime after my husbands decided to re- enlist into the Navy

Reserves. He spent nearly a year in Fallujah, Iraq as a "Seabee". He reenlisted after 9/11/2001.

During his time in Iraq two of our daughters were also in Iraq. Our whole family was so supportive of them all. Both Nurses. One Army (my late husband was also

Army, died during "Desert Storm" 1992) and my other daughter was Air Force. My family has given a lot to our country, and I have given a lot as well.

My settlement with the mesh company was far less than I had expected and counted on. The law firm got 40% and I had to pay to store the mesh for all these years. I also had to pay for incidentals like phone calls, emails, and basically all time spent on my case. It has been a huge eye opener for me. I have never been in a lawsuit before this one. And so what was left over for apparently any entity who had anything to do with my health (XX/XX being one) was offered up. There was $50,000 left. Enough to pay off our home loan. I do not understand why your company would take that from my family and me. We are good, kind, honest, Christian people. My late husband gave it all. My current husband "ran into the fire" for our freedom. My Army daughter gave 10 years and was part of a helicopter mission in Afghanistan, picking up and treating our wounded. My AF daughter ran into shelters every time the "incoming" alarms sounded while in the green zone in Balad. She also cared for Iraqi civilians who were wounded.

Please reconsider taking my money from me. I thought a good insurance company was supposed to help the clients who needed it and make their money on the ones who pay but never need it? I have prayed for this to have a fair ending. And the one thing I really hope to do is to warn all people, especially women, to be sure to ask about surgical mesh. For some reason we trust our doctors literally with our lives and we trust our insurance companies with our premiums. People should be made aware of their right to opt for the old-fashioned way of using the woman's or mans (in the case of hernia repair) existing ligaments to hold things up after a surgery. My mesh was removed in 2014 when I pretty much demanding it to be. Unfortunately, they were unable to access and remove all of it. But even after 12 years my own ligaments are taking the place of the mesh and I pray they will stay strong. My surgeon concurred that the mesh was "contracted and pulling, adhered to my bowel and my urinary bladder, my R ureter was completely scared down" and could have led to me losing a kidney. Because my body attacked the mesh, it also has attacked what was healthy tissue. An Autoimmune response. I now suffer with Hashimoto's Thyroiditis, Leaky Gut Syndrome, Adrenal Insufficiency, Arthritis and more. I would be happy to send copies of my records if you desire.

Please warn the women in your life. This information should be made public. I am willing to bet that like me, there are women living in pain, blaming it on being a woman, having had babies, getting older, etc. I pray you will reconsider something that will be life altering for me. Please do not take the $50,000 that is all I have left.

Sincerely and with gratitude, Diane Ritter-Gardner RN, BSN

I have lost faith in lawyers and in insurance companies. I decided to be done with it. At least I have a newer vehicle with a heated steering wheel. One lawyer did cut his commission for me and I received another small check. I anticipated that my lawsuit would at least cover the salary I would have made working just 24 hours a week as a registered nurse for the 5 years that the mesh was inside of my body. The settlement was not even close.

Also, after hearing how other countries are not standing by women who are desperate for care, it really breaks my heart. I am glad I live in the United States. I feel terrible for the women who have received nothing at all for their hardships. I invested so much of my own time and money tracking down records, while in debilitation pain, staying in touch, keeping the law firm updated, etc., and I do not believe they really cared at all about me.

The whole lawsuit lasted so much longer than I thought and at one time I really considered going into a courtroom. I would have liked to tell my story. I was too ill and too worn out. Then I learned, in the sixth year of my lawsuit, right before my deposition in Philadelphia, that I could not make mention, during my deposition, of the sacral coccygeal Y mesh! This was the mesh which had restricted my life from all basic human functions. I was about to be deposed by a lawyer representing the manufacturer of the mesh. The lawsuit that I had been providing documentation for, driving long distances to get records for, and had put my heart and soul into gaining justice not only for myself but for all women who have been mutilated by this mesh.

The crazy thing I noticed about the legal team representing me was that they chose *not* to depose the doctors who could have helped my case, but instead they deposed at least one doctor who gave false information, who was, coincidentally, the only deposition they offered to share with me. I have no idea what other practitioners they deposed. I know they deposed my entire family, flying lawyers to Maine, which I paid for. If my lawyer had asked me, I could have suggested the three doctors who finally figured out that the mesh was causing all my issues. Obviously, I don't know much about legal issues, but it seems like my law firm did not try to bring in the right people to depose, which could have had a more favorable outcome for me.

Not only had I never been deposed before, but now I had to make sure I did not mention the "monster" that destroyed my life. Sure, the mini-sling was no cake walk. If my husband had not been the extraordinary man that he is, I would have been single by then. Why had they waited six years to tell me that the lawsuit was only for the mini sling? I do not know. And why had they not deposed the doctors who could have done justice to my case?

According to Pub med, in a 2012 study, "The effects of mesh complications caused both physical and emotional pain, in addition to the discomfort of the original pelvic floor dysfunctions, that being dyspareunia (painful intercourse), SUI, irritation and pruritus (itching) of the vaginal and vulva area." This is so true, but the complications turn into life altering, life threatening situations.

There is still mesh in my left sacrum for sure, which aches and "burns" from one side to the other. My surgeon assured me that he was able to get all the mini sling (lawsuit worthy, specifically implanted into our vaginal walls). He was not however able to get all of the Y shaped mesh that is in my sacrum still. He told me that there was a "big blood vessel near the mesh anchor and he could not safely remove it." But he left a bright colored no doubt, polypropylene, suture near it in case I ever needed it removed. More plastic! It is still deep in the bone of my sacrum.

The five pieces of mesh, as seen on the pathology report, are of various sizes and one quite large, up to 3"x 4" approximately. I paid to have this mesh preserved for the entire seven-year lawsuit. Most of the mesh pieces had tissue attached. From the descriptions I have read, I picture the removal to be like taking the string off a Turkey breast once it is cooked As you peel away the string, some won't easily come off and when pulled, tissue is torn away leaving an open area. Once I was convinced that the mesh was my problem, I decided to google the mesh pieces that were listed on my implant log. I was shocked to see one of the mesh kits was available to buy on eBay. For some reason, I just found that odd. Did a big batch of mesh fall off of a truck somewhere, ready to be implanted into someone's body?

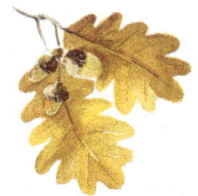

TAPESTRY WITH SHATTERED DREAMS

The ten years that we lived in St. Augustine were meant to fulfill my dreams of a job at a college health clinic where I could teach young people the basics of their health. Another magical dream for me was to live close enough to the beach to go for *a gratifying* walk any time. These dreams were **Stolen** from me as well as so many more.

I am blessed that my girls all adore me. I feel their love and unyielding devotion in my heart. We have been through such devastating times together. I can still feel the love of their dad, their guardian angel.

It has been so difficult to be hurting, *literally* all the time. My girls help my mind go to nicer places. They travel and share their adventures and their fun family times, a few of which we all have shared together. I believe I have had a positive effect on my stepchildren's lives and that we all have shared great family times together. After all, I have been loving their dad with all my heart for 26 years. He has stayed beside me, helped me in any way I have ever asked him or needed him to.

We have survived some tragedies together. One of my daughters tells me now that she completely blocked out when I had brain surgery. She was 16 years old, so I completely understand. My life has been hard on all my immediate family and my close friends. We did have a lot of company in Florida, which at least forced me to get out of bed and get dressed. I apologize for all I may have offended in some of my less compassionate moments, then, now and in the future. *I may as well cover all possibilities.* Thyroid disease is forever!

Life doesn't stop just because
a woman cannot function.

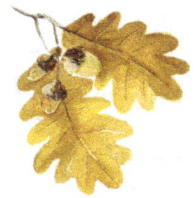

MY STRUGGLE CONTINUES

My husband and I had to go on living during these terrifying sleepless years. We also had other responsibilities.

At this place, in my own ongoing struggle, no diagnosis had been made, I continued with all my own appointments. My husband was the only (helpful) friend I had, and he was very busy.

I saw psychologists for emotional therapy consistently while in Florida and I reunited with my favorite therapist, DD, when we started to "snowbird" in 2013. She was extremely helpful in all areas of my life, but she had a personal issue that took her out of her office for a couple of years. Between 2019 and 2020, up until COVID hit, I saw a different therapist for 24 total visits, using telehealth during COVID because I am still in pain, and I need help getting past all these traumas in my life. This book is currently my therapy.

Seeing and bringing to their attention records from over 20 various practitioners, I was still denied reimbursement for only two years, 2011 and 2012. These were some of the most painful and debilitating years of my fight against surgical mesh and against a healthcare system who had no room in their agenda to give credit where credit was due. Even after the mesh was removed and proven to have damaged my body. I don't understand our social security system at all.

Your Honor,

On Sept 29, 2009, as part of a routine laparoscopic, hysterecto-my surgery, my surgeon chose to use polypropylene mesh (same material used to make PVC pipe) in two areas of my body. This mesh was not approved by the CDC and although I believe there are surgeons still using this "technique," I also read that some of the mesh products were discontinued. The larger mesh (Y shaped) Sacral colpopexy has two shorter ends which when inverted were sewn onto the outside walls of my vagina from the inside of my pelvic cavity "taking the place of my uterus," which had been re-moved. The longer tail end of the "Y" mesh now pointing upward was attached to my sacrum to hold my remaining pelvic organs up and in place. Our sacrum is the lower bone of our spinal column. It is larger than our spinal vertebrae, by approximately four to five times. This bone sits right beside our iliac bone forming our "SI" or sacroiliac joint. Within a few weeks of having the mesh implanted, I started to feel like my pelvis might easily 'break'. I explained this to 30+ practitioners.

I also had developed nausea and a feeling of being poisoned. As my body rejected the PVC mesh, it caused horrific damage to the organs in my pelvic cavity. This coarse mesh substance "ate" its way into my peritoneal cavity leaving my ureter (tube from kid-ney to bladder) completely scarred down to the point where the surgeon had to insert a stent to restore patency. If I had waited and not insisted on removing the mesh, I would most likely have lost a kidney. The mesh was fully embedded and making its way through the vaginal wall from the "outside in" (I am providing the drawing that Dr. M gave me, showing the mesh in red). The mesh also adhered itself to my urinary bladder causing or further ex-pediting the many Urinary Tract Infections that the second mesh was causing. I am sorry this letter is long but it is important be-cause I am concerned for other women (and a few men who may have had hernia repairs using mesh.)

The mesh adhering to my bowel made my chronic constipation even worse. I returned to work as an RN after brain surgery and after my husband of 13 years was tragically killed in a car accident in Germany, where he was stationed during Desert Storm. My cardiologist made note that I had told him I was walking on the beach, as if for pleasure. I did not enjoy the instability of the soft sand or the crab holes, driftwood, rocks and other debris. It was part of an exercise routine. Sitting on anything other than a comfy cushioned seat is uncomfortable and so I try my best to avoid those situations.

I developed several autoimmune reactions in many parts of my body (joint inflammation, especially in Sacro-iliac and finger joints), Hashimoto's thyroiditis (extreme fatigue with both weight loss and weight gain), leaky gut, and a general feeling of being sore and unwell (fibromyalgia) and plantar fasciitis, which is no joke. We walk on our feet every day! Having them be painful holds me back even more. I am unable to work, especially while on medication which I need every day. Being a nurse for 43 years and proud of it, I would not be able to avoid helping someone, a patient or any person should they suddenly start to fall. I would most likely hurt myself and possibly them. But it is in my blood to react. It is instinctual.

There is a "small" amount of mesh left in my sacrum. Since early 2010, I watch every step I take because the slightest amount of drop off on one side or if I misjudge the size of a step will still throw my back into an extremely disabling spasm. I believe this is because the tendons and muscles are stretched out from the five years of pulling by the sacral colpopexy mesh. This is clearly documented in the operative note by Dr. M. According to a recent 60 Minute episode, "polypropylene is not compatible with the human body for long-term use."

None of the various MDs (7), DCs (1) , DOs (3) pain specialists (2), spine specialists (3), physical therapists (6), acupuncturists (1), massage therapists (8), or other holistic healers could help me feel any relief. On most occasions, I felt worse. I have also developed some autoimmune responses and was treated by a Rheumatologist, Dr. Myriam Perez MD, for two and a half years.

After testing me for every possible autoimmune disease and trying many experimental drugs, she diagnosed me with sero-negative inflammatory arthritis and fibromyalgia most likely caused by the polypropylene mesh. I felt like I was being poisoned for all the time the mesh was in me and for months after. Currently, I am taking Lyrica every day as well as ibuprofen, Tylenol, Tramadol and Valium as needed.

He used my own uterine ligaments to replace the large piece of mesh.

Currently and for some time now, I am fighting the scar tissue left behind on my sacrum, which is pulling on my pelvic floor muscles and causing me constant pain and twisting of my lumbar and sacral vertebrae. The autoimmune inflammatory disease affects many joints, especially my sacroiliac and my finger joints. I am continuing pelvic floor PT at home. According to my surgeon, Dr. M, I am one of the unlucky "less than 1% of women who have severe side effects" from pelvic mesh. I can honestly say that I cannot remember the last time that I felt good. It has been since before September of 2009 and I suffered before that with Adenomyosis, among other things. I researched doctors and was not impressed with the Florida surgeons. We had just moved from New England to North Florida. I found a surgeon in Atlanta, Georgia, who was doing hysterectomies by using a laparoscope rather than a big abdominal incision. This surgeon is known for helping women with all kinds of gynecological issues all over the world. My husband happened to be working remotely for his entire employment for this company and it just so happened to have an office in Atlanta which he needed to visit. Since about a month after this "PVC plastic pipe" type of material was implanted in my pelvis, I have had the feeling of being poisoned. I also started having a very unstable feeling in my entire pelvis and low back. It is common-place nowadays for surgeons to use polypropylene mesh to hold up a woman's organs once the uterus, ovaries and fallopian tubes are removed. My surgeon had told me when I asked about complications or side effects, that only less than 1% of women have any problems at all. Unfortunately, I am one of the on lucky less than 1%.

Well, here it is 2:30 AM and I am one of my most frequent places—in my living room in my most comfortable chair with hot tea to hopefully help me sleep.

I wake up in the middle of the night probably 90% of the time. I would really appreciate some financial help from SS. I worked as a nurse for 30 years prior to this surgery. After many hardships in my life including getting hit and almost killed by a car, death of my spouse when our girls were ten, eight and four, brain surgery and now MESH! I feel it is an evil invader of our bodies. So much is around us and in us. But, holding on to hope, my nursing licenses were current in two states for ten years. My Maine license has been active since 1980. Nurses are dedicated people, and I am no exception. I was unable to bend, stand or sit for more than five minutes and the fragile state of my pelvis sent me into spasms that prevented me from giving the patient care necessary. I wish now that I told my story at the first hearing. My disability lawyer is a kind man, and I did not want to go against his advice.

I really appreciate you taking the time to read this letter. I pray that you will have a favorable outcome for me.

Sincerely, Diane Ritter-Gardner RN. BSN.

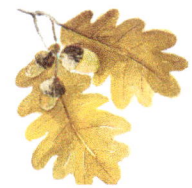

MY LIFE NOW

My days always begin in slow motion with most of my body aching, especially my low back where there is still polypropylene mesh. Many of the autoimmune diseases that were "stirred up" in my body when my immune system tried to fight off the mesh as an invader, are still with me and still I try to remember to have a snack near my bed so that I can take some medication before I must stand up and get moving.

Usually, I start with heat on my back or maybe ice. Heat always feels better but it can increase inflammation if left on for too long. Sometimes I follow heat with ice for about 20 minutes. I find it easier to get dressed on the toilet, especially my lower body. Most days I have a headache due to the increased pressure in the ventricles of my brain. This is an unfortunate symptom that or perhaps ice on my head if I wake up with a headache and breakfast, so I can take my pain meds.

I am working on getting off of one of the sleep meds that I have been on for a very long time. So far, so good. My husband and I are getting ready to meet with an architect so we can build the house of my dreams. This will bring us closer to many of my friends and to St. Joseph's College, where I can get involved with the Silver Sneakers exercise program and other activities as an alumnus.

We got a sweet dog last year. She is seven years old and has created a wonderful bond with my husband and me. He is retired but always busy.

I have been medically retired since 2010, when the mesh started to "talk to me" and limit my abilities. My "job" from then until now has been to find out what was wrong, fix what we could and move forward to be as comfortable, strong and enjoy our five adult kids, four granddaughters, two grandsons and six grand puppies. I guess I have become a "dog person." I must admit that it is nice to be greeted with a wagging tail, excitement and love unconditionally whenever I come home.

Thinking up ways to "play" with our grands is a challenge for me. I am physically limited, but as time goes on, I will improve. That one day years ago when my granddaughter told me one day, "Nana, you are my best friend," really made me appreciate my life. Now, I can't do much better than that. Being a nurse, I will stay connected with the various mesh support groups and pray that I can make a positive difference in many mesh survivor's lives. We have been wronged! But We are warriors. We have to be.

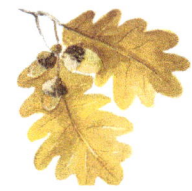

THANK YOU

I want to acknowledge the people who helped make my dream come true.

I am extremely grateful to my loving and ambitious friend Karen who introduced me to Lil, my "editor in chief." Lil B. who has been here for me with guidance and patience from the very first time we chatted. There are other team members, Kirsten, Kristina, Kris are a few I know. I am sure there are others behind the scenes making peoples' rough drafts take on a *published life*, at GWN Publishing. I also send them great thanks for fostering my strong desire to help at least one, but hopefully many women, avoid, manage or have removed any mesh that may be in them or offered to them during a surgery.

The bulk of thanks goes out to my family, who are to me, the real warriors! They have willingly endured my unfortunate circumstance around surgical mesh for 14 years now. Ten of those years living in Florida with only my husband, who, thank God worked from home. I spent many days suffering in silence, not because he or my youngest daughter, who lives in Florida still, were not there for me, but because I too, have my pride. At that point, I felt I should be able to figure out what was wrong. So, I stared at the enormous live oak tree, from my bed every day, reaching roadblocks in my mind. A great amount of recognition goes to my husband and my three daughters who have showed me ever present support and unconditional love from near and afar. Their knowledge and encouragement helped guide me, as well as fueling my persistence in finding out what the heck was devouring every cell in my body, slowly and gradually taking me away, from myself.

I am grateful for the loving relationships our blended family has developed and still have today.

A husband like no other

Everlasting thanks and admiration to my husband Den for staying with me through some of the most devastating years of my life. It is a new year, 2024. The perfect time to dream of a life that is just right for you and me. I want to manage the symptoms and the pain. I am making progress in getting off some medications. During all of the roughest years you never shamed me about taking so many medications. I appreciate that. I know medical stuff isn't for you. I was able to live in peace without worrying that you would question me. Thank you for taking me to appointments and for grocery shopping and cooking and letting me hire a house cleaner and a landscaper among many other unselfish acts. I never felt like doing much and often still don't, but thanks to your encouragement, I did see a few concerts, got to the beach, go downtown St Auggie or wherever *I didn't want to go*. I needed you to get me out. Discussing medical issues have never been for you, at least not willingly, and God knows we have an entourage of medical and dental professionals in our life. I will pray every day that the plastic mesh, still in my bone, never causes me worse pain. That it stays where it is not migrating into another part of my body. I will pray as we are getting older that you never slow down and that you will walk with me for heart health and maybe we can hike again, just small hills are fine. Thank you for standing by me, my husband of 26 years. And thank you for your military service. All 20 years! I have to say that I was entertained and proud of you both, when you gave our daughter, her first salute after

MG (ret)B, commissioned her 2nd LT, United States Army. Thanks for being a great dad to all five of our children.

Loving thanks to Heidi May, my first born, you juggle your life around in circles, while somehow always maintaining stability and love for your family. Pride of country is apparent during Veterans Day ceremonies. Thank you for your service! Thank you for taking care of people on 9D (9 death) as it was known. Although at times you challenge me, I know it is done in love and that you have my best interests at heart. You have only ever pushed me in the right direction. Thank you for supporting me through two surgeries and bringing in your friend M. I have been inspired by your involvement in the community of your children's school and it has given me strength to always do what is right no matter what kind of bull you must put up with. I am so proud of your knowledge and how you continually strive to learn more about life and about raising C & S. I love watching them grow up.

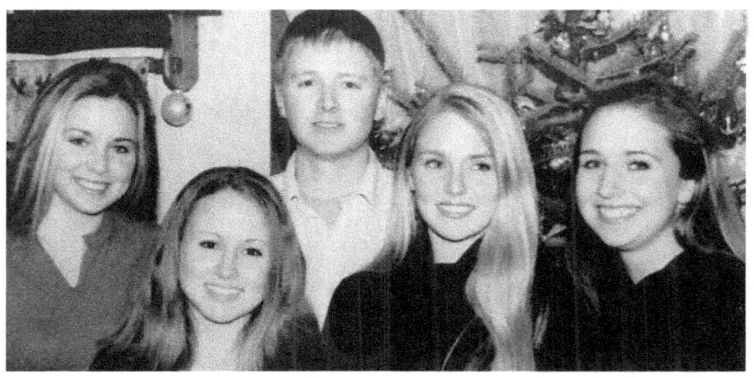

My five children in the early years in the farmhouse.

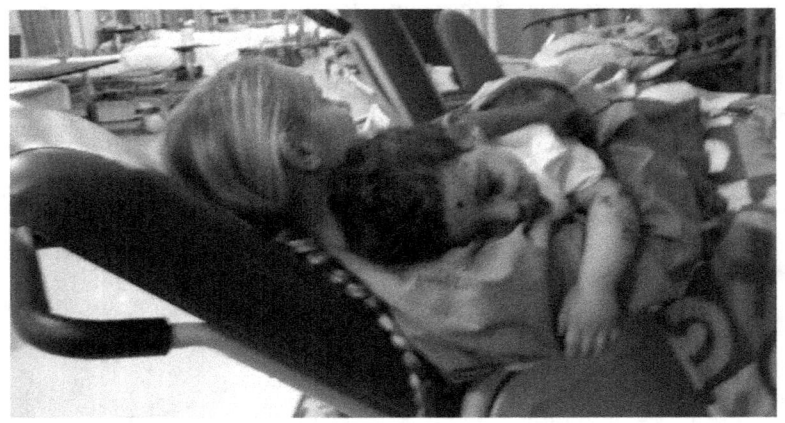

Heidi in Iraq, USAF Nurse Corp

Thanks to my son in law, Jonathan for all you help and support. Much like Heidi, you are strong in mind, will and spirit. You both possess a tender heart, hidden within a suit of armor, shielding your loved ones, me included. Thank you, Jonathan, for standing by me, in my times of need. I respect you fully. I bought the book, "The strong-willed child." when Heidi was a toddler. I bet your mom has it too.

Thank you to my oldest Grandson, Cale, who always greets me with love and maintains a gentleness *around me* that warms my heart. Like your dad, you have a love for animals and baseball. Like your mom, you know what you want, and you go after it. Like me and your mom, you enjoy rocks and gems. I have enjoyed watching you play sports. I get to watch you have fun and get some time away from myself. You and Sage always remember a comfy chair for me, Nana, at your games. You find comfort in moving around, in human touch, or a "pup" will do. I am confident you will go places! I always smile when I see you and Sage, I am not sure where you will venture to in your life yet, Cale, but I know you have the "drive!" Thank you for making me proud. Please never be *too* hard on yourself.

Thank you to my granddaughter, Sage, my sweet "best friend" as you announced one day when you were about four-years-old. You show your love in so many ways but almost always helpful in ways others usually avoid. I remember you scrubbing my steps, (not kidding), folding towels or babysitting a tiny cousin. You are quick to master most things academic or practical. Thank you for trying new things, which brings me joy and thank you for the excitement I see in you when you do a cartwheel. Thank you for being interested in this book, my book. The memories that I share with you, Sage, of playing school and babies, grocery store and making cookies, will always enrich my own fond memories of times with my sister, Auntie Carol. Times of us playing barbies on our bedroom floor, with shoe boxes as beds and baking in our "easy bake oven" *in our closet!* This was not safe, but we didn't know. I appreciate that you and Cale are always thinking of my safety, holding my hand, on uneven surfaces. You protect me, just like your momma and your aunties do. Thanks for being mine.

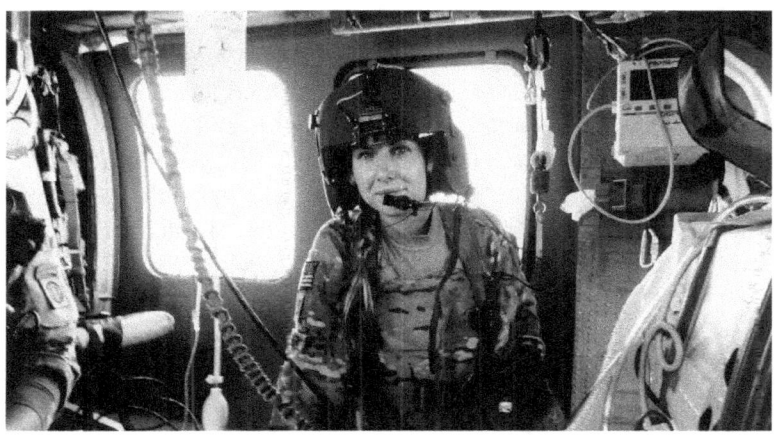

April in Afghanistan, "Dustoff" helicopter mission. USA Army Nurse Corp

Thank you to my middle daughter April. Your positive energy, kindness and gentle nature have made your friends lifelong. I must admit that when you went to "The Stan" to fly with "Dustoff" in Jalabad, it was one of the scariest times of my life. I also know you and I trusted that you would get the job done, retrieve the wounder and protect yourself as necessary. Which you did. Thank you for serving our country! I also appreciated that you checked in with me often. How did Mothers handle wars of our past when snail mail came months after it was written? I am thankful for technology when I see it through the eyes of knowing that my children are a phone call away. I still have a picture in my mind of a room with no ceiling, no privacy from where you could call me. Snail mail by "free post" was so uplifting. There are some pieces of mail in this book somewhere from all my heroes. Thank you for being the middle one, just like your dad. Perhaps a mediator at times? Thank you for knowing that I am here for you always. Becoming a mom to Gavin is a most exemplifying gift for all involved. I know how blessed he is to have you and his dad. I thank your husband Matthew for adoring you. This open expression of his love makes me so happy for you. Thank you, Matt, for always opening your arms in a tender hug for me and for believing in me and this book. Thank you for being helpful and kind.

Gavin, our second grandson, with your dad and your mom, April, as they are, you are blessed. I see you as gentle and loving. Hungry for knowledge. Hanging with dad watching sports and collecting cards. I also love that you collect cool gems and other treasures just like me, your Nana. I believe you are on your way to a dynamic life. Thank you for your smiles and for being my grandson. Thanks to Rose and Dave for sharing you with us so lovingly.

Thank you, Laine, my "youngest," as you so often write. I was the youngest too. We have that in common. I am five years younger than one brother and 10 years younger than the other. I rarely see them; we lead different lifestyles. I forgive them, for being boys, because they are my brothers, because they watched "the three stooges" and because holding on to negative feelings, as you have reminded me, only makes it harder on me. I believe that love forms an unbreakable bond. I am so proud of your perseverance and how you have never given up on your goals like I too have never given up. I love the sisterhood of my three girls. You are a survivor, Laine, a "precious metal," and you have always wanted that for me. I thank God you were nearby to shed some of that "tough skin" my way when I needed it. There were times I wanted to give up, but I knew I couldn't, until I figured out what God wanted for me. Watching you online read a scripture during covid, gave me strength and pride. Your act of courage at that time helped me to keep moving forward. Just knowing you and your husband Lee were close by, gave me comfort. Thank you, Lee, for helping with hurricane clean-up during H-Matthew, and hurricane cooking and physical protection during H-Irma. Also thank you for your support in the Police Force that protects our freedoms. Those acts of kindness are so much appreciated by me.

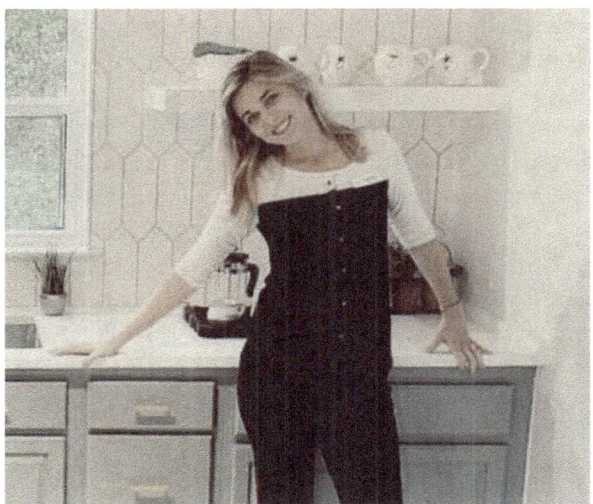

*Elaine, working to help people achieve the "American Dream." My businesswoman.
Mortgage Broker.*

Thanks for all the fun Ryan Heidi, my second granddaughter. And for making me realize how funny kids can be. Ryan, you are smart and a leader in the making. Like your Auntie Heidi, who you are named for. And like your mom, you are a "precious metal," still moldable. With your already present leadership skills, I believe there are wonderful things waiting for you, that is for sure. I believe you will reach for the stars and someday, when you are grown up a little more, your dreams, whatever they turn out to be, will come true. Thank you for being an honest authentic little girl and for being mine.

Thank you to my husband in heaven, Ritter, for watching over me, and our three amazing offspring and the two who hatched in a different nest.

I thank Sarah, my stepdaughter, for your empathetic nature *with me*, and your willingness to take on my burdens when the pressures have been just too much. Thank you for your organizational skills which are a blessing to many, on family trips. Thank you, Tony and Sarah, for the movies on the blowup screen, out in the cold, when a crazy distraction was just what I needed. Thank you for being my fourth daughter and the fourth sister. And thanks for choosing a sweetheart of a husband. You love all pups. And thankfully so does Tony, the famous, "Uncle Tone," as he is called by his nieces and nephews. You are just plain fun to be around, mostly to "whip" the kids and maybe yourself into exhaustion but laughing the whole way through. I know music is your friend, which I would love to hear, but know exists due to the number of guitars that grace your "music room." Thank you for your unconditional friendship and love for me and all our family. If you are in the house, the house is happy! Thank you, Tony, for the "pomp" which brings laughter and excitement for the whole gang.

Thanks to Josh, my Stepson, who has helped me out of a few plumbing emergencies, when Den was in Iraq. I heard a sound like a freight train coming through our 1900 Victorian home here in Maine. I looked around and could not see anything wrong. I opened the door to the garage/basement area and the sound got much louder. Upon reaching the dirt part of the basement, I was met with about four inches of muddy water and then saw the water pouring into the basement. It was not coming from a pipe that I could see. Luckily, I knew how to shut off the main water supply. I'm not sure how you knew where to find the leak, in the pipe, behind the wall? But you found it quickly and cut out a small piece of drywall, and there it was. Thank you also, for making me realize that I was not crazy when I told you that I had polypropylene mesh in my body, and you said, "That is what PVC pipe is made of." Man, that made it real. Thank you for your service to our country.

Rebecca, my daughter in law, thank you for being a great mom, raising two incredibly, sweet, granddaughters. I admire your ability to work where you want because of your experience and credentials. Most of the time you do it all. I know your life is busy and yet if I needed you, I believe you would be there for me. Thank you for our "angelic" third granddaughter, Riley, she will always be in my heart.

Cora, my fourth granddaughter, you have a stern mind, balanced by a cheery disposition. You are a funny, bunny. Curious and smart.

Elise my fifth granddaughter, you are easy going, a little shy at first and then watch out, here she comes. It is so much fun watching you both grow. Thanks for living near us and being a wonderful part of our family.

Thank you, Diane Gail, my sister-in-law. Despite your brain injury, we have shared a lot of fun times. You lived in Florida near us for ten years. At times you required quite a bit of my energy during the mystifying, suffrage that I endured around to the mesh implants. Although these times were physically difficult for me, being your sister gave me hope. Together, we set goals for you, and many were met. You did a lot of fun things like going to Disney, Horseback riding, going to the beach, going on a cruise, you helped yourself and others at the "Center for Living." You also became more independent allowing you to more comfortably interact with people. Helping you gave me a sense of achievement of which I am proud to still offer you, So, Thank you, Di.

My Sissy Carol, we have always been close whether living near or afar. Your unconditional love and support mean the world to me. Thanks for all the "Wild Willys" meet up days, our beach walks in Saint Auggie and our Canada Rides. We will have sister-memories for always. Playing barbies, Christmas mornings, playing in the streets of Somerville, ice skating, fireworks at Foss Park, and so many more. Thank you for taking care of me in the city. Especially when we took the T to Boston. Then the memories of our six girls! How cool is that!! So pleased they are all keeping close. Thank you, Sissy!

My friend Leslie you are my sister in Maine. We have had some wonderful times together and we have many to go. Being around you makes me stronger. I thank you for funneling your pain, to a "hole in the sand," a "dock turns into garden bench," or "a stream can certainly be persuaded to flow opposite of where it wants to go." I can think of so many more projects you have inspired me with. Thank you for loving the outdoors with me, for not giving up on me or yourself. We will hike some more mountains, if it is safe. I am excited to be moving back *home*. Closer to you, so we can get walking and exercising together again. Thank you for helping me proofread part of this book. I am so blessed to have you as my bestie for over 35 years. I'm glad Jay likes me.

My friend Laura. Thank you for being at my side during some of the scariest parts of my life. You are my angel. It will be nice to be nearby again. Once you really retire we can hopefully spend more time together.

My friend Randi. You are one of the strongest women I know. Thanks for your help when I could not clean my own house. I pray every day that you will find a kidney donor, so the trips for dialysis can stop, and you can grow strong again with your two kitties.

I want to thank all the people who I have been in contact with through this whole fiasco! At the risk of leaving someone out, I ask forgiveness upfront. And I doubt my brain will provide 100%. I could play the "brain surgery card?" But instead, I will at least give it a try. My BFF's nearby and far away, are so important to me. Patty and Al, Peggy and Paul, PQ & Chris, Jan & Dana, Sean and Karyn, Lisa & Chip, Gen B and Terry, Alma and Ingrid and many other military friends. Thanks to Gail & Bruce, Nancy, Linda, Martha, Debby, Randi, Gail, Stephanie, and other church and thrift shop friends. Cheryl and Erin, during visits to the cemeteries. I do worry about missing to thank someone, but if you are my friend, you will forgive me and keep in touch.

I am blessed with many other true friends, family and extended family members who have been supportive during these hard years. I have been wanting to write this book for fourteen years. It is a challenge to keep up with everyone, even with social media. Thank you, my nieces Jess, Kris and Sue, also Jenn. Auntie Bunny, Bill P, Garrett, Jane, Colleen, Megs, JT, Sandy & Betsy, Bill and Kasha, Ann and Ed, Joan and Dave. Also, the Maddens, The Gioias, who I enjoy seeing on FB. and Olive's nieces, Liz and Margie. I have been in touch with my dad's extended family, Uncle Bobs daughter, Julie & family. I am thankful for all the people that I keep close to my heart. Friends that I have reconnected with: High school friends: Patrice, Paige, Shawn, Robin and more. Nursing school: Cheryl, Joan, Michelle, Celeste, Marsha and the rest of my class of 15.

I want as much exposure as possible for this book. I am trying to get articles in Magazines. Everyone knows one woman. Maybe that woman is suffering. Maybe she doesn't know why she "feels like hell" but is "putting up with it" or "hanging in there" or "having a hard menopause" or "can't poop" or "peeing all the time "or "always feeling sick" or "always tired". These unspecific and yet common symptoms can mean many things. Please ask if she has had any type of gynecological surgery, if so, she should consider getting her medical records, which *belong to her* and see if there is an implant log that shows use of surgical mesh. If so, there are social media support sites, some gyn surgeon's webpages have descriptions of "mesh failure." There is no lack of information about pelvic mesh or mesh used in hernia repairs today. Thirteen years ago, it was not there. Back then, I looked and found one support group, which I can no longer find. But now, it is clearly advertised as controversial, and there are several support groups involving many countries, and yet, Polypropylene mesh is still being used every day.

Thank you for reading my book. Thank you for helping to spread the word. Let's help people survive mesh together.

ABOUT THE AUTHOR

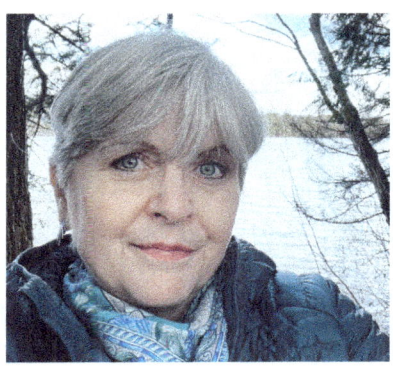

I was born Diane May Bayles in 1959. I married at age 19 in 1979 and became Diane May Ritter. I became a registered nurse in 1980, adding RN to my name. I became a mother in 1982, 1984, and 1987. Tragically, I became a widow in 1992. I remarried in 1997, to become Diane May Ritter-Gardner, RN. I finished my baccalaureate degree in 2000 now becoming Diane May Ritter-Gardner, RN, BSN.

I have enjoyed writing for my own pleasure since I was in high school. My main goal for writing this book is to make as many people as possible, aware of the atrocities, going on *right now*, in the lives and possibly bodies of people who have encountered surgical mesh, are about to be introduced to mesh, or to make some people, like me, aware, that they may already have mesh in their bodies which is making them ill in some way.